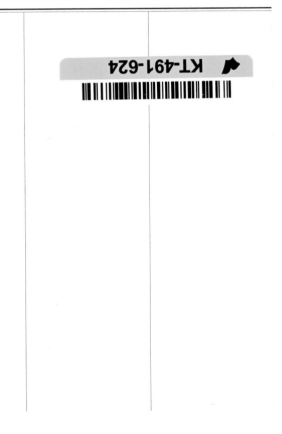

KT-491-624

AUDIT IN ACTION

AUDIT IN ACTION

Edited by

RICHARD SMITH, MB, MFPHM

Editor, British Medical Journal

Articles from the *British Medical Journal*
Published by the British Medical Journal
Tavistock Square, London WC1H 9JR

First published 1992

British Library Cataloguing in Publication Data
Audit in Action

ISBN 0–7279–0317–9

Typeset, printed and bound in Great Britain by
Latimer Trend & Company Ltd, Plymouth

Contents

Page

Introduction xi
RICHARD SMITH, MB, MFPHM, *editor, British Medical Journal, BMA House, Tavistock Square, London WC1H 9JR*

Early perspectives 1

The background 3
Audit in British hospitals 10
Audit in British general practice 18
Acceptability of audit 25
Looking forward to audit 34
CHARLES D SHAW, PHD, *director, Clinical Audit Unit, University of Bristol, Bristol BS8 2PR*

Establishing a framework 41

The role of regional specialty subcommittees in 43
organising audit
C D COLLINS, CHM, *consultant surgeon, chairman regional general surgical subcommittee, Department of Surgery, Taunton and Somerset Hospital, Somerset TA1 5DA*

Organisation of audit in North Derbyshire District 49
Health Authority
RICHARD W McCONNACHIE, FRCP, *formerly consultant physician, coordinator of clinical audit, Department of Medicine, Chesterfield and North Derbyshire Royal Hospital, Calow S44 5BL*

Medical audit data: counting is not enough 57
CYNTHIA LYONS, MPHIL, *research coordinator medical audit*, ROBERT GUMPERT, FRCS, *consultant surgeon, Brighton Health Authority, Brighton General Hospital, Brighton BN2 3EW*

A clinician's guide to setting up audit   68
BRIAN W ELLIS, FRCS, *consultant surgeon, Ashford Hospital, Ashford, Middlesex TW15 3AA*, TOM SENSKY, MRCPSYCH, *vice chairman, district audit advisory committee, Hounslow and Spelthorne Health Authority, Middlesex*

Impact of medical audit advisory groups   78
CLIVE RICHARDS, FRCGP, *regional adviser in general practice audit, South Western Regional Health Authority, Clinical Audit Unit, Department of Epidemiology and Public Health Medicine, University of Bristol, Canynge Hall, Bristol BS8 2PR*

The role of the audit analyst   84
CHRISTINA FIELDING, *clinical audit analyst, Chesterfield and North Derbyshire Royal Hospital, Chesterfield, Derbyshire S44 5BL*

Audit officers: what are they up to?   90
JENNY FIRTH-COZENS, PHD, *regional audit coordinator, Yorkshire Regional Health Authority, Harrogate, Yorkshire, HG1 5AH*, PAMELA VENNING, RGN, *regional audit coordinator, North Western Regional Health Authority, Manchester M60 7LP*

When medical audit starts to count   94
DAVID BOWDEN, FHSM, *managing director, Merritt Health Risk Management, 60 West Street, Brighton BN1 2RB*, KIERAN WALSHE, AHSM, *research coordinator, CASPE Research, Kings Fund, 14 Palace Court, London W2 4HT*

Making audit happen   103

Defining essential data for audit in general practice   105
F DIFFORD, FRCGP, *general practitioner and associate adviser in general practice, 326 Wells Road, Knowle, Bristol BS4 2OJ*

Defining essential hospital data   112
S J NIXON, FRCSED, *consultant surgeon and honorary secretary to Lothian surgical audit subcommittee,*

General Surgical Unit, D Block, Western General Hospital, Edinburgh EH4 2XU

Random review of hospital patient records   116
D A HEATH, FRCP, *consultant physician, Department of Medicine, Queen Elizabeth Hospital, Birmingham B15 2TH*

Criterion based audit   122
CHARLES D SHAW, PHD, *director, Clinical Audit Unit, University of Bristol, Bristol BS8 2PR*

Retrospective review of hospital patient records   129
J G WILLIAMS, FRCP, *director,* M J KINGHAM, BSC, *senior research officer,* J M MORGAN, BSC, *information scientist,* A B DAVIES, MD, *consultant geriatrician, School of Postgraduate Studies in Medical and Health Care, Maes-y-Gwernen Hall, Morriston Hospital, Swansea SA6 6NL*

Problem solving with audit in general practice   136
RICHARD BAKER, MRCGP, *research fellow, General Practice Unit, Department of Epidemiology and Community Medicine, University of Bristol, Bristol BS8 2PR*

Occurrence screening as a method of audit   142
J BENNET, MFCM, *consultant in publich health medicine, Brighton Health Authority, Brighton General Hospital, Brighton BN2 3EW,* K WALSHE, BSC, *research coordinator, CASPE Research, King's Fund, 14 Palace Court, London W2 4HT*

Surveys of patient satisfaction: I—Important general considerations   152
RAY FITZPATRICK, PHD, *university lecturer in medical sociology, Department of Public Health and Primary Care, University of Oxford, Radcliffe Infirmary, Oxford OX2 6HE*

Surveys of patient satisfaction: II—Designing a questionnaire and conducting a survey   160
RAY FITZPATRICK, PHD, *university lecturer in medical sociology, Department of Public Health and Primary*

Care, University of Oxford, Radcliffe Infirmary, Oxford OX2 6HE

Learning and audit   169

Educational aspects of medical audit   170
G F BATSTONE, FRCPATH, *consultant chemical pathologist, Salisbury Pathology Service, General Infirmary, Salisbury SP2 7SX*

A form to help learn and teach about assessing medical audit papers   177
RAJ S BHOPAL, MFPHM, *professor, Division of Epidemiology and Public Health, University of Newcastle upon Tyne, Medical School, Newcastle upon Tyne NE2 4HH*, RICHARD THOMSON, MFPHM, *director of service quality and standards, Northern Regional Health Authority, Newcastle upon Tyne NE6 4PY*

Towards achieving quality   187

Algorithm based improvement of clinical quality   189
STEPHEN C SCHOENBAUM, MD, *deputy medical director,* LAWRENCE K GOTTLIEB, MD, *director, clinical guidelines programme, Harvard Community Health Plan, 10 Brookline Place West, MA 02146, USA*

Variations in hospital admissions and the appropriateness of care: American preoccupations?   198
JOHN P BUNKER, MD, *Clinical Trials Centre, King's College School of Medicine and Dentistry, Rayne Institute, London SE5 9NU*

Arcadia revisited: quality assurance in hospitals in The Netherlands   204
EVERT REERINK, MD, *executive director, CBO, National Organisation for Quality Assurance in Hospitals, PO Box 20064, 3502 LB Utrecht, The Netherlands*

Quality management in the NHS: the doctor's role—I   211
D M BERWICK MD, *associate professor, Harvard Community Health Plan, Boston, Massachusetts 02215, USA*, A ENTHOVEN PHD, *professor, Graduate School of Business, Stanford University, Stanford, California*

94305, USA, J P BUNKER, MD, *visiting professor, CRC
Clinical Trials Centre, King's College School of
Medicine and Dentistry, London SE5 9NU*

Quality management in the NHS: the doctor's role—II   225
D M BERWICK MD, *associate professor, Harvard
Community Health Plan, Boston, Massachusetts 02215,
USA,* A ENTHOVEN PHD, *professor, Graduate School of
Business, Stanford University, Stanford, California
94305, USA,* J P BUNKER, MD, *visiting professor, CRC
Clinical Trials Centre, King's College School of
Medicine and Dentistry, London SE5 9NU*

Introduction

The word audit inspires nobody. It is associated with what the Americans disparagingly call beancounters and summons up thoughts of bureaucracy, control, and money—concepts that have not been seen as important in medicine's effort to improve health. Yet the idea that we should all be trying all the time to improve our performance and our service to patients seems close to the heart of what it is to be a professional. And this is what audit is about. This book, which comprises papers on audit published by the *BMJ* over the past decade, reflects the progress of audit from a marginal activity promoted by a few to a process required of all British doctors that may have profound effects on how medicine is practised in Britain and other countries.

One of the important aspects of the effort to raise quality in health care is that it is a powerful means of bringing together all those working in health services. Doctors and nurses, for instance, have always worked side by side, but they have tended to use different ideas and methods, read different books and journals, and report to different hierarchies. Then, the rise of managers has produced another group with different ways of thinking, and there has been tension between them and health professionals. But the pursuit of quality is something that all the groups can support.

Doctors tend to talk about audit, nurses about quality assurance, and managers about total quality management, but these processes are more similar than dissimilar—and attempts to raise quality demand that the groups come together. Doctors, for instance, setting out to improve the management of patients with hypertension, cannot get far without the input of nurses or managers; nurses will need help from doctors and managers to reduce the incidence of pressure sores; and managers, attempting to reduce waiting times in outpatient clinics, will get nowhere without support from doctors and nurses. This crossing of professional boundaries has been seen as threatening, but those who embark on such projects with other professional groups are more likely to succeed than those who try to do it alone, and they usually find it rewarding.

The pursuit of quality may also profoundly influence health care because of the requirement to think hard about doing the right thing as well as doing the thing right. It is increasingly apparent that many of the activities undertaken by health care workers do not have solid scientific evidence to support them. Many activities are undertaken simply because they have always been undertaken. The first step in audit is usually to think hard about what is being done, and it is this process which throws into sharp relief the question of the effectiveness of interventions. This questioning may be enhanced by the development in the NHS of resource management, whereby clinicians are given responsibility for budgets covering their clinical activities. When clinicians have to decide how to allocate inevitably limited resources they then become very interested in which activities are effective and which are not. Further up the line, the purchasers of the new NHS are also interested in such questions. Doctors and other health workers are understandably made anxious by this intrusion of the concept of cost effectiveness into medicine, but it is in nobody's interest to allocate scarce resources to ineffective activities.

These ways of thinking will inevitably feed through into education, and here again the pursuit of quality will bring change. Students should be made aware of the fragility of the knowledge that is transmitted to them, and the methods of audit and quality assurance should be promoted as lifelong habits. The aim must be to make students aware of the need to search constantly for better ways of practising medicine without undermining their confidence in its practice. The concept of total quality management that "every defect is a treasure" should help: the aim should not be to impart blame for anything that is not done excellently but to find together ways of doing things better. Such a change in belief would have profound consequences within medicine. At the moment there is a tendency to run away from complaints and problems, not least because of the fear of litigation.

Another profound consequence of the pursuit of quality may be to increase the importance of patients. Theoretically the whole of health care is devoted towards improving the health of patients, but few could deny that patients are sometimes relegated to second place in the process. Patients may be woken at 5 am, operated on by a junior doctor in an emergency, given unclear information, and kept waiting for hours in the radiography department, not for their benefit but for the benefit of the smooth running of the institution.

But if patients are the ultimate arbiters of quality then there may be radical shifts in priorities. Two chapters in this book look at the rapidly expanding science of measuring patient satisfaction, and patients' assessments of outcome are one of the more easily measured outcomes as well as being one of the most reliable, meaningful, and reproducible; furthermore, they allow comparisons to be made between widely different sorts of health care.

All this may sound simultaneously frightening and like pie in the sky, but it should not be frightening. Professions need constantly to renew themselves to remain useful, and putting a high premium on quality should be one way for those working in health to enrich themselves. Sometimes the talk of audit and quality assurance is annoyingly vague, and doctors and others are often to be heard saying "Well this is all well and good, but what do we actually do?" Converting the theory and grand statements into reality has been a problem, but that is where this book comes in. It is a practical book that seeks to help doctors and others find their way into audit or the methods of raising quality. It is not the last word on the subject, but I believe that the views and experiences gathered together here will help readers in the practical pursuit of quality and will be relevant for years to come.

RICHARD SMITH
Editor, BMJ

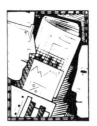

EARLY PERSPECTIVES

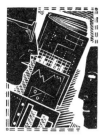

The background

CHARLES D SHAW

Vexation is part of the natural history of medical audit. The question of who should scrutinise clinical work and how has generated a lengthy debate in the United States, Canada, and Australia—and now Britain. The medical profession in these countries has rightly argued that it is inappropriate for the methods evolved in one country for medical audit to be applied unmodified in another. Although there is disagreement and conflicting evidence about audit, certain conclusions have emerged that are common to all these countries and that are now evident in Britain. If the medical profession in Britain fails to take stock of what has been learned about medical audit abroad, the same mistakes will no doubt be made again.

Few subjects evoke as much controversy in the medical profession as medical audit. To some it means assuring clinical standards; to others it is the opposite. Even so, many doctors are coming round to the conclusion that "someone ought to do something about it". What should be done and who should do it would be clearer if there was agreement on what audit is intended to achieve. The widely divergent views on this foster suspicion and distrust of the whole subject by the medical profession, undoubtedly discrediting audit more than it deserves. Even the terminology is forbidding.

Audit by any other name

It is unfortunate that the term "audit"—more usually associated with accountancy—implies numerical review by an outside investigator directed at, among other things, the prevention of fraud. However inappropriately, this connotation has been carried over to what has otherwise been called "medical care evaluation," "clinical and administrative review," "self scrutiny," and a confusing

3

selection of synonyms designed to avoid the misnomer of "medical audit" (table I). Duncan has suggested that "quality assurance" should be applied to the subject in general and "medical audit" to the specific process. By combining any one word from each column in table I in order it is possible to produce 96 phrases that either have been or can be used to mean review of health care.

Various methods of review

Such a cynical simplification conceals important differences between the aims and methods implied in column three of table I, however. Indeed, failure to distinguish between medical audit and monitoring, for example, may account for some of the undeserved disrepute of audit. Doll says that monitoring in the National Health Service implies not only the collection of intelligence to measure progress but also an element of control by health authorities and the Department of Health. While such a method may be appropriate for administration, it is the least acceptable and probably least effective form of audit when applied to the care of individual patients.

Evaluation is defined by the World Health Organisation as "the systematic and scientific process of determining the extent to which an action or set of actions was successful in the achievement of predetermined objectives." Only by using objective research methods can specified patterns of clinical management be related accurately to their effect on clinical outcome. Since most methods of clinical audit rely heavily on the assumption that good care produces good outcomes, audit and evaluation are thus complementary. Although some maintain that these are discrete entities, in practice many audit studies include an element of research.

The Alment Committee report on competence to practise interpreted medical audit as "the sharing by a group of peers of information gained from personal experience and/or medical

TABLE I—Audit by any other name?

Medical	Care	Evaluation
Health	Standards	Assessment
Clinical	Activity	Assurance
Professional	Quality	Audit
		Review
		Monitoring

records in order to assess the care provided to their patients, to improve their own learning, and to contribute to medical knowledge." This is less restrictive in terms of both method and objectives than the American view of Slee (quoted by McWhinney) that medical audit is "the evaluation of the quality of medical care as reflected in medical records."

Sanazaro states the American Medical Association's definition of peer review as the "evaluation by practising physicians of the quality and efficiency of services ordered by other practising physicians." The Welsh working party on medical audit by peer review defined "peers" as "clinicians, all practising in a comparable situation," reflecting the view of the Alment Committee as "doctors who practise in the same specialty and in broadly similar conditions of practice."

These differences are far from academic, and failure to recognise them has caused people in Britain to assume that all the misgivings about audit in North America also apply here. Moreover, a more liberal interpretation will show that to some extent both medical audit and peer review have long been a part of British medical practice.

Internal versus external audit

Internal, clinical medical audit is quite separate from external, non-clinical inspection. The difference between the two concepts may be considered in two dimensions—the extent to which they are external and the extent to which they are non-clinical. At the one extreme of the internal/external dimension is the practitioner reviewing his or her own work and at the other extreme the review of that work by an outside body separated by distance, experience, and values. The clinical/non-clinical spectrum ranges from review by practising clinicians to review by non-medical administrators, community health councils, and lay bodies.

Using this framework, the relations between existing methods for review of health services can be illustrated as in table II. The exact positions of the designations are arguable, but the idea of a continuum is evident. Although not directly relevant to Britain, professional standards review organisation (PSRO) has been included since many of its characteristic shortcomings have been attributed to medical audit in general. The PSRO structure was devised by the United States government primarily to control the

5

TABLE II—Audit of health care

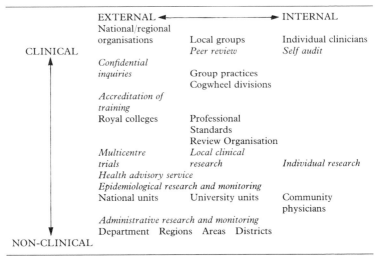

	EXTERNAL ◄————————————► INTERNAL		
	National/regional organisations	Local groups	Individual clinicians
CLINICAL		*Peer review*	*Self audit*
	Confidential inquiries	Group practices	
		Cogwheel divisions	
	Accreditation of training		
	Royal colleges	Professional Standards Review Organisation	
	Multicentre trials	*Local clinical research*	*Individual research*
	Health advisory service		
	Epidemiological research and monitoring		
	National units	University units	Community physicians
	Administrative research and monitoring		
	Department Regions Areas Districts		
NON-CLINICAL			

spiralling cost of government funded health schemes. It was imposed on the medical profession by federal statute, it is not linked to continuing education, and it has the sanction of withholding payment.

Using table II generalisations can be made about what is implied in the review of medical care at either end of the spectrum, internal versus external and clinical versus non-clinical (table III). The external, non-clinical audit may be summarised as statutory and

TABLE III—General characteristics of review mechanisms

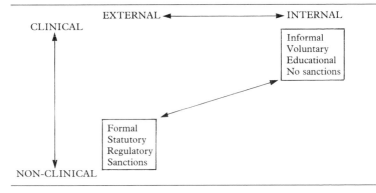

	EXTERNAL ◄————————————► INTERNAL
CLINICAL	
	Informal Voluntary Educational No sanctions
	Formal Statutory Regulatory Sanctions
NON-CLINICAL	

regulatory with implied sanctions. The internal, clinical audit may be summarised as voluntary, educational, and without sanctions.

If "medical audit" was understood in Britain to refer only to self audit and peer review, much confusion and antipathy would be avoided.

Input, process, and outcome

When the decision has been made to review health care, the subject may be approached from many different directions and, in theory, the same conclusions arrived at. But in practice different approaches yield different conclusions, there is no universal means of validating health measures, and even the audit enthusiasts acknowledge that each approach has its weaknesses.

The most quoted model of patient care audit is input, process, and outcome. An example from the manufacturing industry from which the model was borrowed may be helpful: raw materials (*inputs*) are handled in a certain manner (*process*) to produce a finished article (*output*). Each of these elements can be defined in the objective terms of dimensions, numbers, or money as measures for audit. In medicine these elements are often referred to as *structure* (representing resources), *process* (the way in which the resources are applied), and *outcome* (the result of the intervention).

In transferring the industrial model to health care, however, several problems arise. Even if structure and outcome can be measured, the relation between them is variable and badly defined, the quality of care is hard to quantify, and in many conditions the ideal outcome is controversial. It has been suggested, therefore, that patient risk factors and social acceptability should be regarded as separate elements of the model since they appreciably modify the relation between structure and outcome.

Outcome

Ideally an audit of the quality of medical care would focus on the difference between the outcome that is desired and that which actually occurs. In most practice both are hard to define and may occur so long after treatment that many other factors will have intervened to confuse the issue. The concept of "intermediate outcome," such as immunisation take up rates, is a more practical and more sensitive indicator for outcome than the crude but basic measure of mortality, to which studies often resort.

7

Process

Alternatively, audit may focus on the process, such as operation, regimen, or medication, on the assumption that good treatment (as confirmed, for example, by clinical trials) will lead to a good outcome. Some argue that this assumption is invalid since many treatments have never been studied in a controlled setting. And even if they have, are the in vitro results of research applicable to the in vivo reality of everyday practice?

Structure

Audit of structure is even further removed from the outcome of treatment and is, at best, a very indirect measure. Its merit is that resources can be readily measured and the information is accessible. Unfortunately, it is this very convenience (and the absence of better measures) that tempts health administrators to regard norms of input as a substitute for standards of outcome.

Measure of quality of care

Standards, not numerical norms, are the measure of the quality of care, but the medical profession has been reluctant to define standards explicitly. So long as good medicine remains implicit, its evaluation by audit or any other method will remain haphazard.

Bibliography

Calne RY. Surgical self-scrutiny. *Lancet* 1974;ii:1308–9.
Cochrane AL. *Effectiveness and efficiency*. London: Nuffield Provincial Hospitals Trust, 1972.
Committee of enquiry into competence to practise. *Report*. Alment EAJ, chairman. London, 1976.
Doll R. Monitoring the National Health Service. *Proc R Soc Med* 1973;**66**:729–40.
Donabedian A. Evaluating the quality of medical care. *Milbank Mem Fund Q* 1966;**44**,suppl:166–206.
Duncan A. Quality assurance: what now and where next? *Br Med J* 1980;**280**:300–2.
Editorial. Medical audit in general practice. *J R Coll Gen Pract* 1979;**29**:699.
General Medical Services Committee (Wales). *Report of a working party on medical audit by peer review*. Williams DL, chairman. 1975.
Hogarth J. *Glossary of health care terminology*. Copenhagen: World Health Organisation, 1975.
McColl I. Medical audit in British hospital practice. *Br J Hosp Med* 1979;**22**:485–9.
McLachlan G. Introduction and perspective. In: McLachlan G, ed. *A question of quality?* Oxford: Oxford University Press, 1976:3–20.
McWhinney IR. Medical audit in North America. *Br Med J* 1972;ii:277–9.
Matthews MB. Self-assessment programmes and aspects of audit. *J R Coll Physicians Lond* 1979;**3**:139–42.
Mourin K. Audit in general practice. *J R Coll Gen Pract* 1975;**25**:682–3.

Rose JC. Recertification and peer review in the United States. *J R Coll Gen Pract* 1974; **24**:595–7.

Sanazaro PJ. Experience in the U.S.A. *Br Med J* 1974;i:271–4.

Stott NCH, Davis RH. Clinical and administrative review in general practice. *J R Coll Gen Pract* 1975;**25**:888–96.

Wilson LL, Larkins N. Peer review. *Med J Aust* 1977;i,suppl 2:7–24.

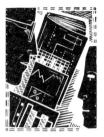

Audit in British hospitals

CHARLES D SHAW

For many reasons acute hospitals appear to be the ideal places to evaluate and develop medical audit in Britain. This is despite the fact that they handle a relatively small and selective proportion of the workload in health care compared with long term care, general practice, and community health.

Most of the pioneering work on audit in North America has focused on hospital care, and many of the problems and possible solutions that have emerged may apply elsewhere. Dr John Porterfield of the American Joint Council on Accreditation of Hospitals has said that hospitals offer the most expensive and most critical form of care, provide the necessary clerical and administrative structure for audit, and deal with the tangible episodes of illness.

In Britain the cogwheel structure of medical advice in hospitals is a more appropriate forum for discussion than is available in many general practices. There are at least some junior medical staff and clerical staff experienced in handling data. Medical records are more uniform and comprehensive, and statistical and diagnostic data are available for inpatients through the Hospital Activity Analysis, the Mental Health Enquiry, and the Hospital In-Patient Enquiry. The purpose and nature of inpatient treatment are easier to define than in other areas of health care, there are fewer patient contacts, and there is more time to examine patients and record information. These advantages reinforce, and are in turn reinforced by, a long teaching tradition.

Formal or informal audit?

Most hospitals have regular meetings to present and discuss selected cases, some concentrating on deaths and complications.

There are doctors who feel that the existing methods of review give adequate assurance of the quality of hospital care, but others argue that regular review should be more formal and include routine performance as well as the management of clinical curiosities. Fernow and McColl offer three reasons in support of this. Firstly, whereas informal audit was adequate in the past when only one clinician was managing a patient, techniques are now needed to audit the performance of the team. Secondly, defining the standards of care would reduce the tendency of external observers to equate efficiency with greater output. And, finally, experimenting with audit now might avoid the pitfalls found in North America.

The following are examples of formal hospital audit: the National Laboratory Quality Control Scheme, the Confidential Enquiry into Maternal Deaths, national studies of deaths associated with anaesthesia (Association of Anaesthetists), deaths among medical inpatients under 50 (Royal College of Physicians), and preoperative chest radiographs (Royal College of Radiologists). Multicentre and national studies are essential for evaluation and for the external audit—that is, audit by organisations outside the hospital or practice—of rare occurrences. But internal audit—that is, self audit and peer review—of daily practice is more appropriate for small, local groups.

Examples of formal audit

Published reports of formal, local audit by peer review are hard to find, in part because they are rarely indexed as such. Some are included here, not because they fulfil the definition but because they show the practicalities of audit. These reports are classified by hospital procedures and units, clinical management, and referrals from general practice. The objectives, methods, and conclusions of the studies are given, but I recommend that the reader refer to the original papers.

Hospital procedures and units

Routine preoperative chest x ray examination (Rees et al, 1976)
Aim To evaluate routine preoperative chest *x* ray examination in non-cardiothoracic surgery.
Method Records of 667 consecutive cases were supplemented, for

11

the latter 152, by questionnaire and analysed with reference to the history, physical examination, and radiological findings.

Findings Patients under 30 years of age represented 16% of the workload but they yielded no significant x ray findings relevant to anaesthesia or surgery: of all significant x ray findings, 54% were due to cardiomegaly and 19% to chronic respiratory disease; 38% had received a chest x ray examination in the past year; 12·5% had received more than the maximum recommended marrow dose.

Conclusions The procedure was being overused and was potentially harmful. Further study was required in order to draft clinical guidelines for its use.

Comment Although this study set out only to evaluate the procedure, it would have been interesting to know, from the viewpoint of audit, whether the findings eventually led to a change in practice. The conclusions were substantially endorsed by a subsequent multicentre study by the Royal College of Radiologists.

Routine chest x ray examination before electroconvulsive therapy (ECT)
(Abramczuk and Rose, 1979)

Aim To evaluate the use of routine chest x ray examination before ECT as a predictor of post-ECT morbidity.

Method Records of consecutive patients attending for two years (total 367) at an ECT clinic were analysed with reference to physical findings, result of x ray examination, and morbidity.

Findings X ray examination gave no extra information relating to risk. One-quarter of the patients apparently had had no physical examination in the month before a course of treatment.

Conclusion The screening procedures, as practised, were ineffective and wasteful; every patient should have a history and physical examination immediately before treatment.

Comment This study shows a common phenomenon in audit— namely, that when routine practice is examined systematically it is often found to differ appreciably from what was assumed to occur.

Perinatal necropsy (Gau, 1977)

Aim To justify postmortem examination of perinatal deaths.

Method The necropsy diagnoses made by one pathologist on 78 cases over three years were compared with the clinical diagnoses.

Findings 11·5% of the necropsy diagnoses differed radically from the clinical diagnoses, and a similar percentage gave added information.

Conclusions Necropsy is a "justifiable intrusion into the sensitivities of medical staff and relatives." It adds confidence to genetic counselling and, as a result of this survey, led to a change in the management of hyaline membrane disease.

Intensive care unit (Tomlin, 1978)

Aim To examine the effectiveness of one intensive care unit (ICU) and its contribution to the workload of other departments.

Method 1718 admissions to the ICU over four years were related to specialty, mortality, and pathology workload.

Findings Mortality in the intensive care unit fell as sophisticated monitoring was introduced for various types of patient. Although mortality within the unit was independent of age (under 70), it correlated closely after discharge from the unit.

Conclusions An inadequate number of beds had resulted in premature discharges and increased mortality. Successful ICU treatment led to a greater nursing workload on general wards. Automatic blood-gas analysis was not only economical but also improved medical care. Earlier introduction of monitoring equipment (delayed for economic reasons) might have saved several lives. Such an audit is valuable for recognising clinical and administrative problems and identifying the effects and priorities of changes in management.

Comment This study shows how audit can be used to generate clinical information on outcomes for more rational planning than is possible basing a study on use of resources (numerical norms of input).

Clinical management

Surgical outpatient follow up (Coggon and Goldacre, 1976)

Aim To assess the value of outpatient follow up after emergency appendicectomy.

Method The records of 351 patients were reviewed retrospectively.

Findings 85% were given follow up outpatient appointments: of those who attended, 12% had complications but only one patient needed to be readmitted. Fewer than half of the patients were seen

13

either by the operating surgeon or his assistant. 94% of readmissions were referred from home by the general practitioner.

Conclusions With the possible exception of patients with complications before discharge, routine follow up could be managed by general practitioners. This would not lessen the variety of teaching material in the outpatient unit but would allow better use of specialist time.

Management of the acute abdomen (Gruer et al, 1977)

Aim To solve some of the problems of diagnosing and managing acute abdominal pain.

Method The initial and final diagnoses in 407 patients seen over six months in a general hospital were compared for general practitioners, accident department staff, and ward medical staff. Guidelines for diagnosis were then issued to hospital staff, and information on diagnostic accuracy was fed back to them. Then, with the help of a community physician, the study was extended to selecting cases for referral by a group of six general practitioners.

Findings The diagnostic accuracy of hospital staff rose from 55 to 77% and the proportion of unnecessary laparotomies fell from 20 to 7%. Of all patients attending the general practitioners with abdominal pain, only 4% were referred to hospital as emergencies.

Conclusions Each participant must be prepared to accept change for improvement and recognise each other's problems. The difficulties of such a project were reduced by a stage by stage approach. Community physicians might contribute to the design of the study and analysis of data.

Comment This audit shows not only how clinical problems are defined but how solutions are found and how their effectiveness can be evaluated.

Accident and emergency radiology (De Lacey, 1976)

Aim To assess the value of radiology to the accident and emergency department.

Method A one year retrospective review of records was combined with a prospective study to define the actual reasons for x ray examination.

Findings Rib injuries were 3% of 10 000 x ray examinations; of these, 13% showed rib fracture and 3% of patients also had a complication (pneumothorax). Each pneumothorax requiring treatment was apparent clinically before radiography.

Conclusions There was minimal clinical value in such an investigation. A frontal chest view to detect complications rather than fractures might be a more economical and effective examination.

Referrals from general practice

Referrals to ear, nose, and throat (ENT) department (Knowles et al, 1979)

Aim To assess ENT training needs for trainees in general practice.

Method The diagnoses by referring general practitioners and consulting specialists were compared for 479 consecutive patients seen over three months.

Findings Referral diagnoses were divided into four discrete groups when analysed according to the degree of agreement with specialist diagnoses, and according to the number of additional diagnoses made by the specialists.

Conclusions Concurrence was poor when diagnosis required skilful examination and interpretive questioning. This suggests a specific need for hospital based specialist training. Such studies are feasible in a small non-teaching district general hospital.

Comment This is tangible evidence of the potential contribution of audit to education.

Appropriateness of referrals (Stott and Davis, 1975)

Aim To enhance the value of referrals to consultants.

Method As part of a regular review programme weekly meetings were held in a teaching group practice to examine each new referral letter. The appropriateness of each letter was discussed in terms of clarity and accuracy of information, choice of specialty, preliminary investigation, and expected response from the specialist. Each referral was reviewed again three months later to compare expected with observed results.

Conclusions The exercise was demanding but educational, demonstrating gaps in knowledge, skills, and communication.

Comment Several studies have examined referrals from general practice as tangible and significant events in patient care.

Experimentation and publication of results

These studies are examples of subjects that can be examined by systematic medical audit, although it may be argued that some are

15

research studies rather than audit. Indeed, since several of the authors could not be described as practising in "the same specialty and broadly similar conditions," as defined by the Committee of Enquiry into Competence to Practise, these studies may be considered to verge on external audit.

Because the form of audit that would be most acceptable to the medical profession would be confidential to the peer group, and because it would be inappropriate to assume that the results of such an audit could be applied to another group in another situation, ultimately there may be no reason to publish accounts of local audit once the principle has been established.

There are many questions about what kinds of audit are workable in Britain. The experience from overseas may answer some, but many require experimentation in Britain and publication of the conclusions. There is no better testing ground than our hospitals.

Bibliography

Abramczuk JA, Rose NM. Pre-anaesthetic assessment and the prevention of post-ECT morbidity. *Br J Psychiatry* 1979;**134**:582–7.

Ashley J, Howlett A, Morris JN. Case-fatality of hyperplasia of the prostate in two teaching and three regional board hospitals. *Lancet* 1971;ii:1308–11.

Brown JM. Why not audit hospital referrals? *J R Coll Gen Pract* 1979;**29**:743.

Coggon D, Goldacre MJ. Outpatient follow-up after appendicectomy. *Lancet* 1976;i:1346–7.

Committee of Enquiry into Competence to Practice. *Report*. Alment EAJ, chairman. London, 1976.

Counihan HE. Evaluation of medical services. *World Hospitals* 1972;Jan:184–6.

De Lacey G. Clinical and economic aspects of the use of x-rays in the accident and emergency department. *Proc R Soc Med* 1976;**69**:758–9.

Dollery C, Bulpitt CJ, Dargie HJ, Leist E. The care of patients with malignant hypertension in London in 1974–5. In: McLachlan G, ed. *A question of quality?* Oxford: Oxford University Press, 1976:37–47.

Dudley HAF. Necessity for surgical audit. *Br Med J* 1974;i:275–7.

Duncan A. Quality assurance: what now and where next? *Br Med J* 1980;**280**:300–2.

Fernow LC, McColl I. The state of British medicine—medical audit. *J R Soc Med* 1978;**71**:787–90.

Fraser RC, Patterson HR, Peacock E. Referrals to hospitals in an East Midlands city—a medical audit. *J R Coll Gen Pract* 1974;**24**:304–19.

Gau G. The ultimate audit. *Br Med J* 1977;i:1580–1.

Gruer R, Gunn AA, Ruxton AM. Medical audit in practice. *Br Med J* 1977;i:957–8.

Hall GH. Medical audit working party's report. *Br Med J* 1979;ii:1603.

Irving M, Temple J. Surgical audit: one year's experience in a teaching hospital. *Br Med J* 1976;ii:746–7.

Knowles JEA, Savory JN, Royle RA, Deacon SP. An audit of ENT referrals assessing training needs for general practitioner trainees. *J R Coll Gen Pract* 1979;**29**:730–2.

McColl I. Observations on the quality of surgical care. In: McLachlan G, ed. *A question of quality?* Oxford: Oxford University Press, 1976:51–61.

McColl I. Monitoring standards of clinical performance. In: *Putting meaning into monitoring*. London: King Edward's Hospital Fund for London, 1979:3–4.

McColl I. Medical audit in British hospital practice. *Br J Hosp Med* 1979;**22**:485–9.

McColl I, Fernow LC, Mackie C, Rendall M. Communication as a method of medical audit. *Lancet* 1976;i:1341–4.

Porterfield JD. What questions need to be answered about peer review? *Med J Aust* 1977;i,suppl 3:31–2.

Rees AM, Roberts CJ, Bliss AS, Evans KT. Routine pre-operative chest radiography in non-cardiopulmonary surgery. *Br Med J* 1976;i:1333–5.

Royal College of Radiologists. Pre-operative chest radiology. *Lancet* 1979;ii:83–6.

Stott NCH, Davis RH. Clinical and administrative review in general practice. *J R Coll Gen Pract* 1975;**25**:888–96.

Tomlin PJ. Intensive care, a medical audit. *Anaesthesia* 1978;**33**:710–5.

Wright HJ, Swinburne K. The general practitioner's use of diagnostic radiology. *J R Soc Med* 1979;**72**:88–94.

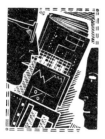

Audit in British general practice

CHARLES D SHAW

During the past 10 years many general practitioners have visibly supported medical audit. Some see audit as a response to the increasing complexity of practice which has led to a greater need for feedback and information. Others see it as a further means of raising the standards of general practice to rank alongside the foundation of the royal college, vocational training schemes, and postgraduate medical centres. In any event, in the second half of the seventies the response to the call for research into medical audit in general practice of the early seventies grew. Much of this work tried to define and suggest solutions to the problems of audit that are peculiar to general practice. Quite apart from the lack of adequate patient records, the virtual absence of reliable information on patterns of practice was a major handicap, as was the lack of clerical help, time, and suitable organisation.

General practice is concerned with people

The overwhelming challenge was (and still is) that the very nature of general practice lends itself even less to objective definition and measurement than its counterpart, the acute hospital. General practice is concerned more with people than with diagnoses, disease, and life threatening events. The objectives take into account social and mental wellbeing and the patient's opinion as much as the clinical response. And the doctor's contribution is as much interpersonal as it is technical. Doney summed up the problem as follows: "If it is difficult to audit the care of diseases, will it ever be possible to audit the care of patients?"

Alternatives for audit

Having recognised the problem, the researchers sought alternative indicators that did not represent the total range of care but that were easier to define. This assumes, as Forsyth and Logan stated, that "it is possible in specific areas and situations to indicate certain concrete things which ought to be done in given circumstances and then to ascertain whether they are being done or not." On this basis some favoured examining "tracer diagnoses"—that is, common, treatable, and definable conditions for which there are generally agreed patterns of management. Some suggested audit of "critical incidents," such as death, complications, and iatrogenic problems. And others analysed patterns of delay in the various stages of patient management. Mourin reviewed these and other approaches to audit in general practice in 1976.

Each approach has its limitations, however, and the usefulness of each depends largely upon the setting in which it is applied in practice. Some of the following studies were part of a continuing programme, others were isolated studies; some included several doctors, or even practices, in peer review, others were one man projects; some were in response to identified problems, others were the byproduct of other inquiries. They give many ideas for audit, but the reader should refer to the original articles.

Audit studies in general practice

Community hospital (Kirk and Lee-Jones, 1976)

Aim To introduce a uniform record suitable for medical audit.

Method A problem oriented medical record was introduced in size A4 for all patients for the joint use of general practitioners, consultants, and nurses. At regular audit meetings attended by doctors and senior nursing staff statistics were reviewed as well as individual cases.

Conclusions The problem oriented record reduced duplication and improved communication but cost money and some confidentiality. Combined audit by nurses, consultants, and all general practitioners allows review of a wide range of clinical problems. Education and appropriate change in practice do follow.

Comment The necessity for adequate, uniform records is emphasised. The decision to include nursing and other staff seems especially appropriate in primary care so long as the intention is to audit practice rather than the practitioner.

Consultation technique (Verby et al, 1979)

Aim To observe the effect of peer review of consultation techniques on experienced general practitioners.

Method Seventeen general practitioners were recorded on videotape during 30 minutes of consultation. Five of them then met weekly to review and discuss each other's recordings, but the other 12 did not. All the doctors were then recorded again and rated according to a validated scale.

Findings The peer review group improved their technique significantly. Higher scores correlated with longer consultations.

Conclusions Experienced doctors can influence change in each other. The five minute appointment system should be re-examined.

Comment Since communication is so critical to the process of care, several authors (Stott and Davis and McColl *et al*) see it as a reflection of the overall quality of care.

Prescribing patterns (Birmingham Research Unit, 1977)

Aim To examine differences in prescribing patterns to establish value judgments on the best use of psychotropic drugs.

Method Four doctors in group practice kept carbon copies of all new prescriptions for one week and repeats for one month. Comparisons were made within the group and with national figures of prescribing rates and therapeutic categories.

Findings Half of the prescribing load (and therefore cost) was for repeat prescriptions. Although new prescriptions for hypnotics and tranquillisers were restricted, repeats were not, leading to long term accumulation.

Conclusions This method provides a simple and effective basis for discussion. It applies not only to other drug groups but also to referrals for diagnostic and therapeutic services. The evolution of internal comparative judgments avoids imposing less appropriate, absolute values. A central confidential databank of comparable analyses would allow baselines appropriate for audit to be established.

Comment Such an objective description of prescribing patterns might be expected to lead to more appropriate therapeutic intervention but Reilly and Patten showed little change on a three week follow up in a similar study, despite group discussion and verbal agreement to change. In another study, Sheldon showed a change in prescribing habits two years after audit but was left with the suspicion that prescriptions were being replaced by referrals for investigation as the final event of consultations.

Clinical management and preventive medicine (Ryan et al, 1979)

Aim To examine various methods of clinical review.

Method Three single handed practitioners working in the same health centre used a simple information system and problem oriented records to analyse aspects of clinical management (minor respiratory illness, urinary tract infection, and prescribing patterns) and preventive medicine (influenza vaccination and recording of blood pressure).

Findings Wide variation in the prescribing of antibiotics and cough mixture in minor respiratory illness invited a consensus on management and repeat of the audit. A previously agreed policy on midstream specimens in urinary tract infections was not being fully applied. Low compliance with an agreed policy to record blood pressure routinely on patients over 20 years of age was particularly noted in women using oral contraceptives and patients with known cardiovascular problems.

Conclusions The auditors were not performing as well in some of their work as they had assumed. The findings were more readily accepted because they were the result of a comparison between subjective expectation and objective observation by themselves rather than by an outside researcher. The experience led to agreement with the recommendations of the Alment Committee of inquiry into competence to practise that such studies are essential in order to achieve a high standard of clinical competence.

Deaths (Ashton et al, 1976)

Aim To explore the value of a peer group in medical audit.

Method As part of a programme of fortnightly meetings over four months, 25 principals reviewed the cases of 55 patients with whom they had been associated and who had died.

Findings Weaknesses were recognised in notes—for example, inadequate or illegible—medications—illogical or unrecorded—and case management—follow up in chronic disease, poor communication with hospital.

Conclusions The method is useful for examining clinical process. Process cannot be audited without adequate records. The weaknesses shown indicate the need for continuing education.

21

Bookings at an obstetric unit (Aylett, 1977)

Aim To retain general practitioner control of bookings at a local obstetric unit.

Method A rotating committee of three general practitioners compared information on each new booking (as given on the booking form and noted by the clinic nurse at the first visit) with the booking policy on contraindications previously agreed by the medical staff committee. If a booking seemed inappropriate, a note giving reasons was sent to the doctor concerned, but there was no direct sanction.

Findings Bookings of inappropriate high risk cases diminished rapidly over two years.

Conclusion Peer review is adequate to effect a change in practice without applying compulsion.

Comment This also shows how prospective audit using locally agreed criteria can resolve a very real problem. Retrospective audit has also been used by Shapland and Marsh to evaluate booking policies of individual doctors and remote obstetric units.

Chronic disease (Doney, 1976)

Aim To examine the process of medical care of a chronic disease (diabetes) in general practice.

Method The records of 119 known diabetics in an eight person practice were analysed.

Findings Before diagnosis, classic symptoms but no urine test were recorded in 16% of patients. Roughly one quarter of the patients attended the general practitioner, one quarter attended a consultant clinic, and half had no regular supervision. Only 12% were controlled on diet alone.

Conclusions Recording of diabetic control and regular follow up was poor. Relatively low complication rates may have reflected a low detection rate. The current family practitioner committee record card is a deterrent to long term follow up of chronic disease. More data for comparison are needed about patients in the community rather than in hospital clinics.

Comment Problems of follow up and recording of patients with diabetes were also noted by Kratky, but allegations of similar inadequacies in the care of epilepsy were refuted in an audit by Zander *et al*. On the basis of existing prevalence data, Wilson concluded that many hypertensive patients were not detected in his practice.

Delay patterns (Jenkins, 1978)

Aim To evaluate delay patterns as an index of medical care in general practice.

Method Seven general practitioners pooled data on 55 new cases of neoplastic disease over one year. For each case delay was analysed as that attributed to the patient and that attributed to medical services. An estimate was also made of the proportion of the latter delay that was inevitable had circumstances been ideal.

Findings Diagnostic delay was generally reasonable but there was evidently room for improvement in some cases.

Conclusions The index was probably not an adequate measure of the total quality of care, but none the less it showed specific and remediable elements of the process. The exercise raised the doctors' index of suspicion for new cases of cancer.

Comment In a similar study that related presenting symptoms to delay in diagnosis and treatment, Macadam suggested that research into clusters of symptoms and risk factors to enable early referral of appropriate cases would be more rewarding than research into cancer cures in hospital. In an earlier study of diagnostic delay, Hodgkin pointed out the implications of the method for directing the education of both patients and doctors.

In these studies in general practice many different methods were used by individuals and by groups of doctors. Some of the studies were specific research projects and two used computer analysis, but the concepts can be applied to most practices. The people who participated found the exercise educational, many unexpectedly gaining insight into their own style of medicine. Some doctors argue that audit should not be done at all unless it can be shown to improve the outcome of care. Such solid evidence is difficult to obtain from relatively small numbers of patients, even in large group practices, without doing multi-group studies which would destroy the local and internal nature of the audit they seek to evaluate.

Audit should probably focus on the process of care, but on the condition that the information generated is used to bring about appropriate change and that the change is then evaluated to show that it was effective. Perhaps this is the next step for audit in general practice.

Bibliography

Acheson HWK. Medical audit and general practice. *Lancet* 1975;i:511–3.
Acheson HWK. Why standards? *J R Coll Gen Pract* 1978;**28**:692–5.

Ashton J, Oliver G, Grant A, Taylor GK. An audit of deaths in general practice. *Update* 1976;**12**:1019–22.

Aylett M. Bookings at a general practitioner obstetric unit: an exercise in peer review. *Br Med J* 1977;ii:28–9.

Buck C, Fry J, Irvine DH. A framework for good primary medical care—the measurement and achievement of quality. *J R Coll Gen Pract* 1974;**24**:599–604.

Birmingham Research Unit of the Royal College of General Practitioners. Self-evaluation in general practice. *J R Coll Gen Pract* 1977;**27**:265–70.

Capstick I. Need for pilot studies in general practice. *Br Med J* 1974;i:278–9.

Committee of enquiry into competence to practise. *Report.* Alment EAJ, chairman. London, 1976.

Dollery C, Bulpitt CJ, Dargie HJ, Leist E. The care of patients with malignant hypertension in London in 1974–5. In: McLachlan G, ed. *A question of quality?* Oxford: Oxford University Press, 1976:37–47.

Donabedian A. The quality of medical care: a concept in search of a definition. *J Fam Pract* 1979;**9**:277–84.

Doney BJ. An audit of the care of diabetics in a group practice. *J R Coll Gen Pract* 1976; **26**:734–42.

Anonymous. Down with audit. *Practitioner* 1979;**223**:427–8.

Forsyth G, Logan RFL. *Towards a measure of medical care.* London: Nuffield Provincial Hospitals Trust, 1962.

General Medical Services Committee (Wales). *Report of a working party on medical audit by peer review.* Williams DL, chairman. 1975.

Hodgkin GK. Evaluating the doctor's work. *J R Coll Gen Pract* 1973;**23**:759.

Jenkins S. Diagnostic delay in neoplastic diseases. *J R Coll Gen Pract* 1978;**28**:724–8.

Johnson R. A method of evaluating treatment in general practice. *J R Coll Gen Pract* 1974;**24**:832–6.

Johnson R. Medical audit. *Lancet* 1975;i:679.

Kirk C, Lee-Jones M. Medical records, medical audit and community hospitals. *J R Coll Gen Pract* 1976;**26**:143–6.

Kratky AP. An audit of the care of diabetics in one general practice. *J R Coll Gen Pract* 1977;**27**:536–43.

Macadam DB. A study in general practice of the symptoms and delay patterns in the diagnosis of gastro-intestinal cancer. *J R Coll Gen Pract* 1979;**29**:723–9.

McColl I, Fernow LC, Mackie C, Rendall M. Communication as a method of medical audit. *Lancet* 1976;i:1341–4.

McDowell I, Martini CJM. Problems and new directions in the evaluation of primary care. *Int J Epidemiol* 1976;**5**:247–50.

Mansfield P. The study and evaluation of general practice. *J R Coll Gen Pract* 1973;**23**:887–94.

Marsh GN. Obstetric audit of a general practice. *Br Med J* 1977;ii:1004–6.

Metcalfe DHH. Medical audit. *Br Med J* 1974;iii:327.

Mourin K. Audit in general practice. *J R Coll Gen Pract* 1975;**25**:682–3.

Mourin K. Auditing and evaluation in general practice. *J R Coll Gen Pract* 1976;**26**:726–33.

Reilly PM, Patten MP. An audit of prescribing by peer review. *J R Coll Gen Pract* 1978; **28**:525–30.

Ryan MP, Buchan IC, Buckley EG. Medical audit—a preliminary report from general practice. *J R Coll Gen Pract* 1979;**29**:719–22.

Shapland DE. Extended role for general practitioners in obstetrics? A medical audit. *Br Med J* 1979;i:1199–200.

Sheldon MG. Self-audit of prescribing habits and clinical care in general practice. *J R Coll Gen Pract* 1979;**29**:703–11.

Stevens JL. Quality of care in general practice: can it be assessed? *J R Coll Gen Pract* 1977;**27**:455–66.

Stott NCH, Davis RH. Clinical and administrative review in general practice. *J R Coll Gen Pract* 1975;**25**:888–96.

Stott NCH, Davis RH. Medical audit. *Lancet* 1975;i:679.

Verby JE, Holden P, Davis RH. Peer review of consultations in primary care: the use of audiovisual recordings. *Br Med J* 1979;i:1686–8.

Wilson JB. An audit of hypertension in a rural practice. *Practitioner* 1978;**220**:689–92.

Zander LI, Graham H, Morrell DC, Fenwick P. Audit of care for epileptics in a general practice. *Br Med J* 1979;ii:1035.

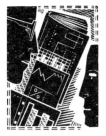

Acceptability of audit

CHARLES D SHAW

Arguments about how acceptable and workable medical audit is in Britain are based as much on conjecture as on practical evidence, owing both to the lack of experience in Britain and to the natural fertility of folklore. Moreover, because of the many different meanings ascribed to audit and the various methods used, generalisations cannot usefully be made.

The debate on the acceptability of audit focuses on three questions: how is it controlled? what does it cost? does it work? The last question, probably the most difficult one, carries the assumption that certain objectives can be fulfilled and that these may then be used to measure the effectiveness of audit. There is disagreement, however, even about the objectives.

Objectives of medical audit

It is generally agreed that education is the main purpose of medical audit. The Birmingham Research Unit of the Royal College of General Practitioners describes this more specifically: "curiosity, organised by [medical audit] is basically a process of self-education." Planning may be considered a second purpose and include information on how resources are used. A third objective of audit is to evaluate medical care, a fourth to add to medical knowledge, and a fifth to forestall, by anticipatory diplomacy, external audit being imposed on the medical profession from outside.

Some authors believe that the first objective of medical audit is to improve standards of care. It is extremely difficult to show such an effect, however, except in terms of changes in the process of care. To assume that an improvement in care follows automatically from changes in the way care is given is an attractive argument. Indeed, this assumption is inherent, therefore unproved, in many informal activities of postgraduate medical education.

These objectives are generally acceptable to the profession and are not greatly contested. That the profession has a duty to review its own work is implicit in medical practice: so implicit that, according to Dudley (1975), we are embarrassed to talk about it. The divisive issue is whether more formal audit should replace the traditional forms of review.

Dilemma

In its evidence to the Royal Commission on the NHS, the BMA said, "We are not convinced of the need for further supervision of a qualified doctor's standard of care." The commission subsequently reported, "We are not convinced that the professions regard the introduction of medical audit and peer review with a proper sense of urgency." As stated in editorials in the *British Medical Journal* (1976) and the *Practitioner* (1979), some would rely on the "innate sensitivity of the profession" to maintain standards rather than the "chopping block of medical audit."

Others argue that isolated debate and conventional review have no effect on how medicine is practised, and that formal analysis and feedback are necessary to prevent the same mistakes recurring. Moreover, there is evidence that traditional continuing medical education is unlikely to resolve existing problems. A study by Ashbaugh and McKean of 5400 patients' records in the United States suggested that 94% of the deficiencies were failures of performance rather than of knowledge.

But such evidence may not apply here in Britain. Even if it did the complex systems of audit in the United States would not. The motivation for audit and the structure of health care are quite different in Britain. The now dominant professional standards review organisation (PSRO) was set up in the United States to control increases in costs, fees, and unnecessary surgery. In Britain the problem is to get necessary surgery done. The open access for medical staff in most hospitals in the United States allows a wide variety of doctors to see inpatients, whereas in Britain the traditional referral system from general practitioners, a salaried, hierarchical hospital staff, and a "professional bureaucracy," ensure that, for example, all patients for surgery are supervised by fully qualified surgeons and anaesthetists. (But this should not encourage the common misbelief that doctors in the United States are totally free agents; on the contrary they work under more explicit regulations than British doctors.) Naish pointed out that audit facilitates control in the United States where the distances between places are so vast, and Matthews suggested that the popularity of audit is inversely proportional to reverence for authority.

Characteristic attitudes

Although Matthews offered his hypothesis to explain the different attitudes toward audit between Britain and the United States, it may also explain differences within these countries. Metcalfe has said that young doctors show a greater enthusiasm for audit than established doctors. This may reflect irreverence for established practice, a greater need for reassurance, or the effect of continuous assessment during training. This generation gap is also shown by newly qualified doctors relying on laboratory rather than clinical data, which sometimes causes problems in agreeing on the appropriate management of a patient. Hall took the point further by suggesting that terms such as peer review, monitoring, and assessment were "intoxicating to the sado-masochistic academics and the new breed of MRCGPs."

Effectiveness of audit

Effective audit may be regarded as a three part cycle of setting standards, evaluating care, and modifying practice in the light of the evaluation (figure). Many audits fail in the last stage because there is no formal feedback of information and no formal decision to remedy the deficiencies that are discovered. Without feedback and remedy "orphan data" merely accumulate. This has been the fate of many PSRO studies, and Nelson says that this is because the clinicians whose work is being audited reject the standards used for evaluation because they did not help to formulate them—a problem inherent in any system of audit that is not internal. Brook and Williams showed that by adding educational feedback to the PSRO system these same audits were effective in modifying behaviour. Williamson, however, had previously shown the opposite: that doctors who had failed to respond to unexpectedly

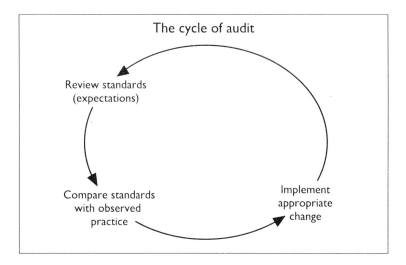

abnormal screening results performed no better after taking part in a specially designed awareness programme.

In general the studies of McSherry, Nelson, and Kessner in the United States, that have been quoted as showing that audit does not work, referred to the specific shortcomings of a system that is unlikely to reach Britain and not to audit itself. Brook and Avery recognise that some of these failings are not sufficiently great to justify abandoning the concept altogether, even in the United States.

McSherry concluded that audit failed to identify educational needs at Cornell, but studies in Canada and in Britain suggest that this is not a universal rule. Experience in Britain has likewise shown the value of audit in planning and evaluating medical services, though there is conflicting evidence on the effectiveness of audit in influencing change. Some studies showed that audit was not followed by an appropriate modification in clinical practice, while others showed that it was. In particular, Gruer *et al* noted that after starting audit in a surgical department the clinical diagnostic accuracy of acute abdominal pain improved and the number of negative laparotomies decreased.

In short, the evidence that medical audit can be effective is not overwhelming, but it suggests that audit has a brighter future in Britain than PSRO has in the United States.

Control of audit

Even if there is some reassurance that audit can be justified in terms of effectiveness, a major source of anxiety remains: who will be affected, and who will be in control? Doctors are concerned that the profession's authority, already diluted by pressure from team management, administrators, and patients, will be further scrutinised by outsiders until medicine is "practised in a goldfish bowl," as Stevens aptly put it.

Customer audit is unpopular

The public is becoming increasingly interested in medical care, and Klein argues that those who use public resources should be accountable to the public for the way in which they dispose of those resources. Many doctors feel that if audit is inevitable it should be organised by the profession before someone else fills the administrative vacuum, but some do not agree that audit is inevitable. In either event, customer audit does not seem popular, nor does the possibility of legal intervention and the "fearsomely destructive weapon of negligence," that Johnson warns of. If medical audit gave proof of a deviation from an explicit set of criteria for patient management, could this be used as legal evidence against a doctor?

Centrally imposed audit is misconceived

"The Government, who pay the piper, will insist that the tune is at least audible," but a State-run audit would be unacceptable. Similarly, there is concern that a review system set up in good faith by the profession might subsequently be taken over as an external audit or that the information generated might be abused.

A centrally imposed audit would be misconceived. This is in part because there are few validated national standards of management; in part because (as has been shown in the United States) external audit has little effect on education or change; and also because audit would take on the image of bureaucracy. External audit has a limited application—for example, in quality control of clinical laboratories and in confidential inquiries into maternal mortality. With such exceptions the role of central administrative bodies and the royal colleges should be to provide assistance, advice, and information for audit. Clinicians might also turn for help to community physicians, though they have so far shown little enthusiasm for that role.

Local audit may lead to rigid standards

If a successful case is made for leaving audit to small, local groups this too would place some restriction on clinical freedom, even if only at the very margins of clinical reason. Some fear that using explicit criteria would lead to a rigid orthodoxy of elitist standards that would ossify clinical practice and stifle innovation. Others would welcome more uniform behaviour, or they at least believe that an individual should defend the choice of a different approach. And, if clinical freedom is as much a right of the patient as of the doctor this freedom would not justify doctors rejecting a step towards evaluating patient management.

Mandatory audit leads to sanctions

The final question on control is whether audit should be mandatory and whether sanctions should be imposed on those doctors found wanting. Such policing would probably be counter-productive, but it is also recognised that voluntary mechanisms of education are most used by those who least need them. It has therefore been suggested that items such as payments for seniority and vocational training should be dependent on evidence from audit that the objectives of these schemes, rather than their process, have been fulfilled. The Royal Commission on the NHS suggested that hospital training posts should be approved only in departments where an "acceptable method of evaluating care has been instituted."

Cost of audit

The prospect of any innovation that might encourage defensive medicine and overinvestigation in order to comply with explicit standards is unwelcome in the NHS but is a much less realistic hazard than in the United States. Indeed there is some evidence that audit would reduce unnecessary procedures in Britain and provide a more rational basis for the allocation of the limited resources in the NHS. Implementing the remedies suggested by audit usually requires reorganisation—for example, of communications or follow up—rather than expenditure. However, the process of audit uses up resources: any method of audit will require the clinicians' time, even if much of the workload is carried by secretarial or clerical staff. The cost of internal audit in Britain would be nowhere near the amount quoted for running the complex American PSRO structure, but even if "a good system of medical audit is worth any number of postgraduate courses," as McWhinney suggests, this may amount to discouragement.

In 1976–7 the cost of running the PSRO programme was variously stated as having been 66, 70, and 90 million dollars—roughly 0·05% of the 150 billion dollar cost of the entire health system in the United States. McSherry calculated the average cost of one audit in one large teaching hospital at just under 5000 dollars in 1976. This contrasts with the combined experience of several hospitals in the Niagara Peninsula of Canada in 1977 where an average audit study required 23 hours of medical records staff time. In Britain the Birmingham Research Unit estimated that one audit had required 17 hours of secretarial time at a marginal cost to the practice of less than £10 in 1975. The amount of time required and the costs were expected to drop in both cases as systems became better established.

The limited published experience of audit in Britain suggests that it would be less costly and more effective than PSRO has been in the United States. But this reassurance alone will do little to dispel underlying doubts about the wider implications in practice. When the medical profession has ensured its own authority over audit then it may be easier to accept.

Bibliography

Abramczuk JA, Rose NM. Pre-anaesthetic assessment and the prevention of post-ECT morbidity. *Br J Psychiatry* 1979;**134**:582–7.

Acheson HWK. Medical audit and general practice. *Lancet* 1975;i:511–3.

Anonymous. Medical audit. *Lancet* 1978;i:1166.

Ashbaugh DG, McKean RS. The philosophy and use of audit. *JAMA* 1976;**236**:1485–8.

Ashton J, Oliver G, Grant A, Taylor GK. An audit of deaths in general practice. *Update* 1976;**12**:1019–22.

Aylett M. Bookings at a general practitioner obstetric unit: an exercise in peer review. *Br Med J* 1977;ii:28–9.

Birmingham Research Unit of the Royal College of General Practitioners. Self-evaluation in general practice. *J R Coll Gen Pract* 1977;**27**:265–70.

British Medical Association. Evidence of Council to the Royal Commission on the National Health Service. *Br Med J* 1977;i:299–334.

Brook RH, Avery AD. Quality assurance mechanisms in the United States. In: McLachlan G, ed. *A question of quality?* Oxford: Oxford University Press, 1976:221–52.

Brook RH, Williams KN. Effect of medical care review on the use of injections. *Ann Intern Med* 1976;**85**:509–15.

Capstick I. Need for pilot studies in general practice. *Br Med J* 1974;i:278–9.

Chisholm JW. Medical audit. *Br Med J* 1979;ii:143.

Clark MR, MacIntyre KA. Patient care appraisal as a guide for the design of continuing medical education: 10 years' experience in the Maritime provinces. *Can Med Assoc J* 1978;**118**:131–8.

Committee of enquiry into competence to practise. *Report*. Alment EAJ, chairman. London, 1976.

Counihan HE. Evaluation of medical services. *World Hospitals* 1972;Jan:184–6.

Coggan D, Goldacre MJ. Outpatient follow-up after appendicectomy. *Lancet* 1976;i:1346–7.

Devitt JE. Does continuing medical education by peer review really work? *Can Med Assoc J* 1973;**108**:1279–81.

De Lacey G. Clinical and economic aspects of the use of *x*-rays in the accident and emergency department. *Proc R Soc Med* 1976;**69**:758–9.

Duncan A. Quality assurance: what now and where next? *Br Med J* 1980;**280**:300–2.

Dudley HAF. Necessity for surgical audit. *Br Med J* 1974;i:275–7.

Dudley HAF. Can we audit cost-effectively? *Br Med J* 1974;iii:274–9.

Dudley HAF. Audit and the pathologist. *Proc R Soc Med* 1975;**68**:634–7.

Editorial. Towards medical audit. *Br Med J* 1974;i:255.

Editorial. Controlling quality. *Br Med J* 1974;iii:704.

Editorial. Audit of audit. *Lancet* 1976;ii:453.

Editorial. Audit again. *Br Med J* 1976;ii:714.

Editorial. Separating the sheep from the goats. *Br Med J* 1976;ii:1218.

Editorial. Quality control of laboratories—or of pathologists? *Br Med J* 1977;i:1180.

Editorial. Medical audit and continuing education. *Br Med J* 1978;ii:156.

Editorial. Medical audit now. *Br J Hosp Med* 1979;**22**:421.

Editorial. Medical audit in general practice. *J R Coll Gen Pract* 1979;**29**:699.

Editorial. Down with audit. *Practitioner* 1979;**223**:427–8.

Editorial. Medical audit in general practice. *Lancet* 1980;i:23–4.

Gau G. The ultimate audit. *Br Med J* 1977;i:1580–1.

General Medical Services Committee (Wales). *Report of a working party on medical audit by peer review*. 1975.

Gerber A. Medical audit. *Lancet* 1975;i:1086.

Gruer R, Gunn AA, Ruxton AM. Medical audit in practice. *Br Med J* 1977;i:957–8.

Hall GH. Say "no" to audit. *World Medicine* 1979;**14**:21–2.

Hodgkin GK. Evaluating the doctor's work. *J R Coll Gen Pract* 1973;**23**:759–67.

Horsley S. Medical audit. *Br Med J* 1979;ii:143.

Irvine D. Contemporary professional practice. In: McLachlan G, ed. *A question of quality?* Oxford: Oxford University Press, 1976:65–96.

Johnson R. Medical audit. *Lancet* 1975;i:679.

Joint working party on the organisation of medical work in hospitals. *Second report*. London: HMSO, 1972.

Kessner DM. Quality assessment and assurance: early signs of cognitive dissonance. *N Engl J Med* 1978;**298**:381–6.

Kirk C, Lee-Jones M. Medical records, medical audit and community hospitals. *J R Coll Gen Pract* 1976;**26**:143–6.

Klein R. An alternative approach to audit. *Br Med J* 1976;ii:597–8.

Knowles JEA, Savory JN, Royle RA, Deacon SP. An audit of ENT referrals assessing training needs for general practice trainees. *J R Coll Gen Pract* 1979;**29**:730–2.

McColl I. Medical audit in British hospital practice. *Br J Hosp Med* 1979;**22**:485–9.

McColl I. Monitoring standards of clinical performance. In: *Putting meaning into monitoring*. London: King Edward's Hospital Fund for London, 1979:3–6.

McColl I, Fernow LC, Mackie C, Rendall M. Communication as a method of medical audit. *Lancet* 1976;i:1341–4.

McLachlan G. Monitoring health services. *Int J Epidemiol* 1976;**5**:83–6.

McSherry CK. Quality assurance: the cost of utilization review and the educational value of audit in a university hospital. *Surgery* 1976;**80**:122–9.

McWhinney IR. Medical audit in North America. *Br Med J* 1972;ii:277–9.

Matthews MB. Self-assessment programmes and aspects of audit. *J R Coll Physicians Lond* 1979;**3**:139–42.

Metcalfe DHH. Medical audit. *Br Med J* 1974;iii:327.

Mourin K. Auditing and evaluation in general practice. *J R Coll Gen Pract* 1976;**26**:726–33.

Murray JH, Swanson AL, Knauf C. Canadian Council on Hospital Accreditation project shows clinical appraisal can be satisfying. *Can Med Assoc J* 1977;**116**:200–5.

Naish JM. Medical audit. *Br Med J* 1974;i:514–5.

Nelson AR. Orphan data and the unclosed loop: a dilemma in PSRO and medical audit. *N Engl J Med* 1976;**295**:617–9.

Porterfield J. Peer review—answers to some of the questions posed. *Med J Aust* 1977;i,suppl 3:29–33.

Rees AM, Roberts CJ, Bligh AS, Evans KT. Routine pre-operative chest radiography in non-cardiopulmonary surgery. *Br Med J* 1976;i:1333–5.

Reilly PM, Patten MP. An audit of prescribing by peer review. *J R Coll Gen Pract* 1978;**28**:525–30.

Royal College of Surgeons of England. Evidence to the Royal Commission on the National Health Service. London, 1977:part II.

Royal Commission on the National Health Service. Measuring and controlling quality. In: *Report of the Royal Commission*. London: HMSO, 1979:173–7.

Ryan MP, Buchan IC, Buckley EG. Medical audit—a preliminary report from general practice. *J R Coll Gen Pract* 1979;**29**:719–22.

Secretary of State for Social Services. A sound management structure. In: *National Health Service reorganisation: England*. London: HMSO, 1972.

Shackman R. Medical audit. *Br Med J* 1974;i:388–9.

Sheldon MG. Self-audit of prescribing habits and clinical care in general practice. *J R Coll Gen Pract* 1979;**29**:703–11.

Smart GA. Monitoring in medicine. *J R Coll Physicians Lond* 1975;**9**:355–70.

Stevens JL. Quality of care in general practice: can it be assessed? *J R Coll Gen Pract* 1977;**27**:455–66.

Stott NCH, Davis RH. Clinical and administrative review in general practice. *J R Coll Gen Pract* 1975;**25**:888–96.

Thould AK. Medical audit necessary, but rigidity greatest danger. *Br Med J* 1974;i:279–80.

Tomlin PJ. Intensive care, a medical audit. *Anaesthesia* 1978;**33**:710–5.

Verby JE, Holden P, Davis RH. Peer review of consultations in primary care: the use of audio visual recordings. *Br Med J* 1979;i:1686–8.

Williamson JD. Quality control, medical audit and the general practitioner. *J R Coll Gen Pract* 1973;**23**:697–706.

Williamson JW, Alexander M, Miller GE. Continuing education and patient care research. *JAMA* 1967;**201**:118–22.

Wilson LL, Larkins N. Peer review. *Med J Aust* 1977;i,suppl 2:7–24.

Looking forward to audit

CHARLES D SHAW

Consumer organisations, community health councils, and other thoughtful lay bodies are increasing the pressure for accountability of health care, and this is echoed by cries from within the medical profession that the profession should be seen to examine its own work critically. Many doctors view audit not with delight but with resignation and the hope that, if it is inevitable, something good will come of it. Perhaps it is the price we pay for being in the profession with the fastest rate of change.

Few formal medical bodies during the past five years have failed to endorse the concept of audit by the profession. The third report of the Joint Working Party on the Organisation of Medical Work in Hospitals avoided the specific phrase medical audit, but voluntary peer review was explicitly supported by the Alment Committee on competence to practise, the working party of the Welsh General Medical Services Committee, and most recently the Royal Commission on the National Health Service. In their evidence to the royal commission the Royal Colleges of Physicians of London, Surgeons of England, and General Practitioners all advocated some form of audit as a method of education or evaluation. In contrast the BMA was tepid in its support, but it was urged at the conference of senior hospital staff in 1978 and at the Annual Representative Meeting in 1979 that practical approaches to audit be explored. So it looks as if the issue is no longer whether medical audit will become established in Britain but what form it will take. And this equally fertile issue will no doubt provide medical journals with editorial pabulum for several years.

Authors who have faced the problems of implementing audit have drawn up guidelines, based on their experience, on its purpose and practice. These vary in emphasis, but factors common to the different sources are as follows:

34

purpose—should be educational and shown to be relevant to patient care;

control—should be by clinical peers and participation should be voluntary;

standards—should be set locally by participating clinicians;

method—should be non-threatening, interesting, objective, and repeatable (for follow up);

resources—should be cheap and simple and cause minimal disturbance to clinical work;

records—adequate clinical content and retrieval systems are essential.

Although most of these points have been covered earlier in this series, little has been included about the choice of method or the practical needs of audit.

Topics for audit

The longstanding question of whether to focus on outcome of care or on the process of care is still unresolved but has recently been summarised by McColl (1979). Another point for debate is whether audit should be performed on practice, practitioner, or health care in general. Although they provide food for philosophy, these issues have little practical application since the individual elements cannot be realistically separated from each other. Different approaches are appropriate to different problems.

An ideal subject for audit would be a common, well defined, clinically significant diagnosis or treatment where management has a clear effect on outcome. It is obvious that few subjects are ideal and certainly do not represent the whole range of clinical practice, but several close approximations may be suggested (see tables I and II). Though not all aspects of medicine lend themselves to audit, this does not diminish the value of what is learned from

TABLE I—Some topics appropriate for audit in acute hospitals

Use of antibiotics	Appendicectomy
Blood transfusions	Cholecystectomy
Cardiac arrest	Inguinal hernia
Hypertension	Massive gastrointestinal bleeding
Anaemia	Pre-anaesthetic assessment
Urinary tract infection	Obstetric flying squad calls
Bacterial pneumonia	Induction of labour
Paediatric gastroenteritis	

TABLE II—Some topics appropriate for audit in general practice

Hypertension	Pyrexia of unknown origin
Diabetes	Surveillance of elderly at home
Thyroid disease	Backache
Leg ulcers	Urinary tract infection
Otitis media	Depression

those that do. Apart from studies in general practice and of inpatient care in acute hospitals, there is little published experience in Britain. The audit of long term hospital care, community health, and outpatient care (including casualty) presents different problems requiring different solutions.

Information and records

One issue on which the practitioners and philosophers are universally agreed is that audit quickly shows how inadequate the average traditional medical record is for explaining what happened to patients and why. This is perhaps most evident in chronic illness managed by various team members in primary care. Some remedies are the use of A4 filing, flow sheets, and problem oriented records. But changing record systems is sufficiently expensive, time consuming, and daunting that many doctors would first need to be convinced that the upheaval would be rewarded by improved patient care. As a compromise, problem lists and team participation—two main features of problem oriented records—can be applied to traditional records but are not essential to audit.

Another requirement for audit is a system of retrieving the records of patients with a given diagnosis, treatment, or procedure. In hospitals the Hospital Activity Analysis and Mental Health Enquiry may be supplemented by registers kept in individual departments for inpatients, but comparable sources for outpatients are limited. Similar problems in general practice have been met by using diagnostic registers, colour tabulations, and feature card systems.

Information about practice patterns and about the evaluation of traditional processes of patient management requires knowledge that can only be built up by a central collection of data and by controlled research.

36

Choosing a method of audit

Examples of several approaches were given earlier in this series in relation to hospitals and general practice. Some of those were based on informal, subjective reviews of sample cases—a low key, straightforward approach that may encourage participants to break the ice and gain confidence in peer review. Experience in North America, however, has shown the limitations of this method. Because the method is subjective, small groups tend to avoid drawing conclusions or recommending actions that are likely to lead to confrontations with colleagues. In addition, by taking samples only a small proportion of cases can be reviewed, which is costly in terms of the doctors' time and gives only a limited view of patterns of practice.

Criterion audit

Such problems led to the development of "criterion audit," which is now the preferred method in the United States and Canada since it can be applied to any group of patients with some characteristic in common. Having chosen a topic for review, the participating doctors agree on a limited number of tangible elements that they consider to be critical to the process and outcome of management. For example, an audit of the treatment of patients with pneumonia in hospital might include referring to specific elements of diagnosis, treatment, and resolution and defining undesired complications.

These criteria are explicitly formulated so they can be applied by medical records staff to individual patient notes and recorded as either present or absent. In this way, 30 to 50 records can be reviewed, but only a small minority, which for some reason vary from the agreed criteria, are examined by the clinicians themselves. A large proportion of the records showing variation are then seen to be justified clinically, leaving only a few that are considered by the group to show specific defects. On this basis the group can make appropriate recommendations for future management.

On first sight this approach seems to be unnecessarily complicated and restrictive, but in practice it is not and it has many advantages in addition to avoiding the potential problems of subjective, selective audit. Discussing the essential criteria before the audit is performed reduces any perceived need for self-justification and is in itself an education since it requires agreement on issues that may otherwise be considered too basic to be debated. However, since such explicit criteria have been condemned in Britain for producing rigid conformity in patient management, it must be emphasised that their purpose is merely to cull records for clinical review. They do not provide a prescription for managing patients.

Like committees, an audit that does not produce explicit conclusions and explicit recommendations for action is useless. This formal approach also permits the same study to be repeated later so that direct comparisons can be made to show whether the recommended actions were actually effective in resolving the previous weaknesses.

Clerical staff already assist in tabulating data in primary care, but criterion audit relies heavily on medical records staff in hospitals as well. In the Canadian equivalent of district hospitals it is becoming usual for one member of the records staff to be trained and employed for this purpose. This "records analyst" also handles data for the equivalent of the Hospital Activity Analysis, which provides much of the information for case retrieval.

In Britain, where there is no equivalent to the records analyst, health authorities must recognise that formal audit cannot be established without the help of adequately staffed records departments. Some consolation from the implications of the cost may come from the analogy that in industry it has long been accepted that "quality control" is an integral part of the budget.

Finally, it should be stressed that the role of medical records staff in criterion audit is to collect and tabulate data from clinical records, using the criteria defined by the doctors, and not to exercise clinical judgment.

Introduction of audit

In Australia, the United States, and Canada the development of audit has been fostered in hospitals by national systems of hospital accreditation. These non-governmental bodies not only visit all types of hospitals every two to three years, but they also publish guidelines on good practice in running hospitals. They are thus well placed to advise and assist in the development of audit. Although in Britain the Health Advisory Service could fulfil part of this role, encouragement would come most appropriately from the royal colleges and faculties in coordinating pilot studies and seminars. At the local level assistance in establishing audit should come from community physicians and, because the primary role of audit is to educate, from postgraduate tutors. Community physicians and postgraduate tutors should take part only at the request of clinicians who seek to implement audit, and their role must be to advise rather than to perform the audit.

A medical organisation for carrying out audit and for implementing and following up recommendations for change is also needed. The cogwheel system was intended for this purpose, and doctors in group practice or health centres have an advantage. But special problems are faced by doctors isolated by distance or specialty and they may require coordination by local medical committees or regional departments.

The requirements for audit may be summarised as information, resources, and willingness to participate. There is little that is new about the concept of review, except the terminology and, more visibly, the formal methods. The principal ingredient is one of attitude—as an editorial in the *Lancet* recently stated, "Without a willing spirit of enquiry, audit is worthless."

Bibliography

Birmingham Research Unit of the Royal College of General Practitioners. Self-evaluation in general practice. *J R Coll Gen Pract* 1977;27:265–70.

British Medical Association. Evidence of Council to the Royal Commission on the National Health Service. *Br Med J* 1977;i:299–334.

British Medical Association. Annual Representatives Meeting, 1979. Medical audit: ARM calls for practical recommendations. *Br Med J* 1979;ii:143.

Buck C, Fry J, Irvine DH. A framework for good primary medical care—the measurement and achievement of quality. *J R Coll Gen Pract* 1974;24:599–604.

Canadian Council on Hospital Accreditation. *Guide de Contrôle Médical.* Toronto, 1976.

Clark MR, MacIntyre KA. Patient care appraisal as a guide for the design of continuing medical education. *Can Med Assoc J* 1978;118:131–8.

Committee of enquiry into competence to practise. *Report.* Alment EAJ, chairman. London, 1976.

Conference of senior hospital staff, 1978. Medical audit working party's report. *Br Med J* 1979;ii:1603.

Dudley HAF. Necessity for surgical audit. *Br Med J* 1974;i:275–7.

Editorial. Controlling quality. *Br Med J* 1974;iii:704.

Editorial. Medical audit in general practice. *Lancet* 1980;i:23–4.

Fernow LC, McColl I. The state of British medicine—medical audit. *J R Soc Med* 1978;71:787–90.

General Medical Services Committee (Wales). *Report of a working party on medical audit by peer review.* 1975.

Irvine D. Contemporary professional practice. In: McLachlan G, ed. *A question of quality?* Oxford: Oxford University Press, 1976:65–96.

Irving M, Temple J. Surgical audit: one year's experience in a teaching hospital. *Br Med J* 1976;ii:746–7.

Johnson R. Medical audit. *Lancet* 1975;i:679.

Joint working party on the organisation of medical work in hospitals. *Third report.* London: HMSO, 1974.

Kirk C, Lee-Jones M. Medical records, medical audit and community hospitals. *J R Coll Gen Pract* 1976;**26**:143–6.

McColl I. Observations on the quality of surgical care. In: McLachlan G, ed. *A question of quality?* Oxford: Oxford University Press 1976:51–61.

McColl I. Medical audit in British hospital practice. *Br J Hosp Med* 1979;**22**:485–9.

McColl I, Fernow LC, Mackie C, Rendall M. Communication as a method of medical audit. *Lancet* 1976;i:1341–4.

McDowell I, Martini CJM. Problems and new directions in the evaluation of primary care. *Int J Epidemiol* 1976;**5**:247–50.

Mourin K. Audit in general practice. *J R Coll Gen Pract* 1975;**25**:682–3.

Mourin K. Auditing and evaluation in general practice. *J R Coll Gen Pract* 1976;**26**:726–33.

Murray JH, Swanson AL, Knauf C. Canadian Council on Hospital Accreditation project shows clinical appraisal can be satisfying. *Can Med Assoc J* 1977;**166**:200–5.

Reilly PM, Patten MP. An audit of prescribing by peer review. *J R Coll Gen Pract* 1978; **28**:525–30.

Royal College of General Practitioners. Evidence to the Royal Commission on the NHS. *J R Coll Gen Pract* 1977;**27**:197–206.

Royal College of Physicians of London. *Evidence to the Royal Commission on the National Health Service.* London, 1977.

Royal College of Surgeons of England. *Evidence to the Royal Commission on the National Health Service.* London, 1977:part II.

Royal Commission on the National Health Service. Measuring and controlling quality. In: *Report of the Royal Commission.* London: HMSO, 1979:173–7.

Ryan MP, Buchan IC, Buckley EG. Medical audit—a preliminary report from general practice. *J R Coll Gen Pract* 1979;**29**:719–22.

Sheldon MG. Self-audit of prescribing habits and clinical care in general practice. *J R Coll Gen Pract* 1979;**29**:703–11.

Stevens JL. Quality of care in general practice: can it be assessed? *J R Coll Gen Pract* 1977;**27**:455–66.

Wilson LL, Larkins N. Peer review. *Med J Aust* 1977;i,suppl 2:7–24.

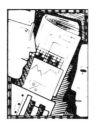

ESTABLISHING A FRAMEWORK

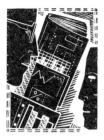

The role of regional specialty subcommittees in organising audit

C D COLLINS

Hospital medical staff are now prepared to talk about, discuss, and criticise audit, but as yet little has been achieved, except by individual enthusiasts. For audit to be properly conducted and effective a considerable change is needed in consultants' attitudes. Such change requires guidance and encouragement; the royal colleges and faculties have offered general guidelines and the government has provided a timetable, requiring all consultants to be involved in medical audit by 1991.[1] It is, however, a big step from the receipt of such guidelines to detailed implementation of audit by individual consultants. There are few clinicians, even in the larger specialties, with an enthusiasm for conducting audit, and many specialties have too few members to permit a meaningful comparison of activity. Audit within specialties is therefore probably most effectively coordinated, if not organised, on a regional basis, as has been shown over the past few years by the Lothian surgical audit.

Regional specialist advisory committees can bridge the gap between college guidelines and individual district or specialist audit activities. To be effective such committees must assume and be given by their colleagues responsibility as the peer group from whom guidance and leadership may be obtained in the setting up, conduct, and practice of audit. The organisation of such committees is important, with regard to their membership and their relation with each other, regional management, and individual consultants. One example of how this might be achieved is currently in practice in the South Western region.

The South Western regional hospital medical advisory committee is composed of a consultant nominated by each of the 11 districts and selected, as far as possible, from different specialties, the postgraduate dean, and a university representative, currently the professor of community medicine. The regional medical officer and his senior medical assistant attend regularly, and the regional manager attends when possible. The committee has called on skill from the King's Fund to assist it and its subcommittees in developing medical audit; it assumed this responsibility in the region almost a year before the white paper was published and acts as the regional audit committee. It circulated its guidelines *The Regional Approach to Medical Audit* in June 1989. Through the participation of the regional manager, and access, therefore, to the management network, it is possible to bring pressure on district and unit managements to provide facilities and support necessary for the proper conduct of audit.

In the south west the regional primary health care committee links general practitioners in the district into a regional audit framework and provides guidance and coordination to the district audit committees. It also has an important role in promoting dialogue between both sides of the hospital-primary care interface and fostering an understanding by each of the perceptions and priorities of the other; these are not always obvious and may stimulate the identification of certain useful outcome indicators. The regional hospital medical advisory committee has been concerned with (a) development of software for audit; (b) establishing the extent of support of administrative and clerical staff for the clinical teams; (c) arranging for consultants to have sufficient sessional time to carry out audit; (d) organising training for doctors concerned with setting up and initiating audit; and (e) setting up regional arrangements for medical audit in specialties with only a few consultants in each district, through appropriate subcommittees. The role of regional specialty subcommittees varies with the number of consultants in each specialty. Those of the larger clinical specialties, such as general surgery, medicine, and trauma and orthopaedics, monitor, encourage, and coordinate the district audit activities. The smaller subcommittees either act as specialist audit committees in their own right or coordinate the activities of two or three subregional groups of consultants.

Audit in general surgery

There are currently more general surgeons in the South Western region undertaking systematic audit than any other specialists. Many have several years' experience which can be used in the organisation and practice of audit in their districts. For maximum effect the membership of a regional general surgical subcommittee should include a member from each district, preferably with management, educational, or audit responsibilities or experience, an expert audit adviser, a health care evaluator, a representative of the postgraduate dean or university, and a senior member of regional management plus secretarial support. A committee so constituted might then be able to gain the confidence of all the consultants in the specialty and offer guidance and specific proposals on the conduct of audit, both of the process and of the outcome of surgery. Such a committee must deal with several problems.

Attitude of consultants—Consultants' attitudes towards audit might be encouraged and developed by a combination of carrot and stick; for surgeons the stick has been supplied by the Royal College of Surgeons, which suggested that recognition of the training of junior surgeons might be conditional on evidence that

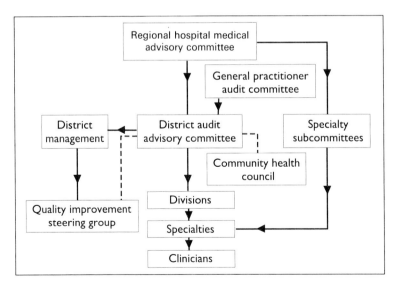

Regional audit structure

effective audit meetings have taken place with all surgical staff present and that appropriate records of such meetings have been kept.[2] The carrot might be the adjustment of a clinically overcommitted timetable to permit time for the disciplines of self assessment, discussion, and self education implicit in the conduct of audit. The regional medical advisory committee may best coordinate the particular requirements for time, technology, and administrative assistance and make clear statements on these matters so that pressure can be applied on district and unit managements to make the necessary resources available.

Agreement on data capture—Many surgeons conduct either complete or partial audit with a desktop microcomputer, a card index system, or some other personal system. The regional advisory committee has urged that the development of stand alone clinical computer audit systems should not be supported and recommends that microcomputers should be linked directly to the hospital patient administration system. One such system is the medical data index being developed for the South Western region in Taunton, which forms the basis of a clinical workstation and not only provides an almost limitless memory for audit purposes but also produces discharge summaries for the general practitioners and accurate coding for transfer to the hospital system. Because all districts in the region use the same DEC-VAX mainframe computer systems the possibility exists for future regional analyses of surgical activity.

Agreement on coding—There is an urgent need for national agreement but because the International Classification of Diseases (ninth revision) diagnostic coding and Office of Population Censuses and Surveys (fourth edition) operation coding will probably be adopted as the standards these are the two systems encouraged in the region. If other coding systems are already in use, as for example in Lothian, then it would seem wise to develop a software package which could translate the existing individualised codes into the adopted codes.

Agreement on severity and complexity coding—Current NHS performance indicators permit comparison of the number of patient episodes, operations, discharges and deaths, and the resources used but take no account of the clinical severity of the patient's condition or the complexity of the procedures undertaken. For audit it is essential to agree on both. The clinical severity index used in the confidential inquiry into perioperative deaths was that of the American Society of Anesthesiologists. This is currently used in the South Western regional pilot medical data index scheme. The American Medisgrps system is currently being evaluated in Bristol. Operative complexity has usually been assessed using the British United Provident Association (BUPA) scale, although a modification of the new BMA scale might become more generally acceptable. Regional, if not national, agreement on these two quality factors is being sought.

Assessment of surgical outcome—Much of the current medical reporting is devoted to that of individual short or long term follow up studies, many of which would be greatly strengthened by expansion to include different units in the region. Such coordination may be organised through the regional specialty subcommittees. Similarly standardised assessments of outcome may be agreed with the help of health care evaluation skills, academic input, and administrative support.

Identification and organisation of supradistrict specialist surgical services—The confidential inquiry into perioperative deaths and the Lothian audit have indicated the benefit to patients of allocating the care of less common conditions to experienced specialists. Districts cannot expect to offer the highest quality of care in every sphere of surgical activity. The strengths of individual surgical units for certain specialist activities should therefore be identified and recognised by the regional committees so that recommendations may be made for resources to be set aside to foster and develop suitable skill. Examples include renal transplantation, hepatic resection surgery and possibly oesophageal surgery, laser treatment, and the development of specialised endoscopic procedures. Such activities could be centred in any district general hospital where the specialised interest and skills of consultants are available.

Regional surgical audit report—A regional surgical audit report might comprise a brief amalgamation of individual district audit reports, and would promote the enthusiasm and the industry put into audit by providing a goal for individual district surgical audit committees. Effective changes in practice in one or other district would be highlighted and might then be coordinated into formulating regional management advice. Alternatively, conflicts in practice between districts might become a subject for audit by the regional specialist subcommittee itself.

All these audit functions require administrative, secretarial, and technological resources, which must be made available if the laudable aims of medical audit are to be achieved.

In conclusion, regional specialist advisory committees have an important part to play in the development and conduct of medical audit and have a special advantage in that consultants generally feel accountable to the region as their contract holder and will more readily accept advice from the region than that emanating from the district or unit, which they think is often guided more by resource implication than by the desire for improved clinical service. They may call on the resources of the health authority and the university, the royal colleges, and on specialist advice for help in coordinating and formulating policies and reports. By setting timetables and posing specific questions regional specialty subcommittees may help to implement the policies of the royal colleges and the Department of Health on the practice of medical audit.

1 Secretaries of State for Health, Wales, Northern Ireland, and Scotland. *Working for patients.* London: HMSO, 1989. (Cmd 555.)
2 Royal College of Surgeons of England. *Guidelines to clinical audit in surgical practice.* London: RCS, 1989.

Organisation of audit in North Derbyshire District Health Authority

RONALD W McCONNACHIE

In 1987 Trent Regional Health Authority decided that each district health authority should set up a quality assurance programme. The chairman and district general manager of North Derbyshire District Health Authority visited each specialty group to discuss quality assurance and ask for its cooperation. Medical audit is an essential part of quality assurance, and I was asked, as chairman of the medical staff committee, to provide a discussion document giving my view on how medical audit might be implemented throughout the district. The document explained the philosophy and process of audit and gave definitions and examples. It also suggested a structure suitable for districtwide audit, and this was debated by the consultant medical staff committee. Most consultants were enthusiastic about audit but expressed concern regarding confidentiality, lack of an accurate diagnostic index, difficulties in specialties with fewer than three consultants, and problems with allocating time for audit. I subsequently visited each specialty group to discuss the problems, and we eventually agreed on objectives, structure of the audit, and allocation of time, as follows.

Objectives of audit

Our objectives were:
• To develop a voluntary system of audit throughout the district that included all consultants and junior staff

49

- To have a structured audit
- To appoint a senior clinician as coordinator
- That each specialty group would set up its own methods of audit but would be helped by the coordinator when necessary.

The first specialty groups started audit in January 1988, and by the autumn of 1989 regular audit had been established in all major specialties. Only three departments, all with fewer than three consultants, had been unable to take part. These were the ear, nose, and throat; accident and emergency; and dermatology departments. The ear, nose, and throat and dermatology departments now actively participate in interdistrict audit. Although initially having problems finding adequate time and medical cover to come to meetings, the accident and emergency department has undertaken project work with the aid of the audit department and organised weekly dinnertime meetings. Because these are amalgamated into one set of monthly minutes, all staff can attend at some time.

Structure of audit

The figure shows the structure of the audit. The audit coordinator reports to the district audit committee which in turn comes under the jurisdiction of the hospital medical advisory committee. He has access to the unit general managers and to the district general managers and, if it were ever necessary, direct access to the district health authority.

The coordinator was appointed in 1987 and his duties are:

- To coordinate the various participating specialty groups
- To act as liaison officer—for example, to arrange time available for audit meetings and secretarial help and to discuss with management recommendations for audit when they entail a change of policy or extra resources
- To collate information from all sources of audit and act accordingly
- To monitor action recommended by the various groups
- To provide and monitor statistics including performance indicators and to request comments
- To arrange interdisciplinary meetings
- To review and circulate published reports on audit
- To suggest subjects for discussion to the groups
- To advise on what to audit and how to do so, when requested

- Membership of the district audit committee, the postgraduate education committee (with regard to the educational needs for audit), and the regional hospital board's audit steering group
- To review complaints and untoward incidents
- To facilitate audit for smaller specialties that collaborate with other district health authorities in the region.

Audit activity

In view of the many terms relating to audit we decided to define three types of audit activity and the staff who should be involved:

Medical audit—synonymous with peer review. This involves only doctors and may be either self audit, when one consultant and his or her junior staff take part, or unit audit, when all consultants and junior staff from that specialty are involved.

Clinical audit—that is, anything to do with direct patient care. In addition to doctors, nurses and paramedical staff are asked to attend. This type of audit is common in the surgical specialties.

Resources to support audit

1987 A coordinator appointed with two sessions weekly, increasing to four sessions from 1990

March 1988 A research assistant appointed with four sessions per week to provide the administrative back up for all audit, to help with research projects, to advise on computer analysis, to coordinate secretarial help for audit groups, and to provide statistical data and their interpretation

1990 A full time clerk and a full time secretary to be appointed to support the coordinator and all specialty groups

1991 Full time audit analyst to organise and collate all data collected. Part time support manager whose responsibilities include the formulation of the annual report. Full time audit assistant to provide aid to project work and secretarial assistance to the chairman.

Medical management audit—for example, the management of inpatients or of outpatient waiting lists and admission or discharge policies for a ward. Secretarial and administrative staff are included in addition to doctors, nurses, and paramedical staff.

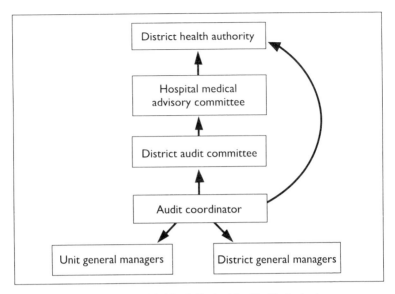

Structured audit as performed in North Derbyshire Health Authority

Audit methods

The time allocated to audit was agreed with the district general manager, and currently the major specialties meet once monthly, usually for two and a half hours. The surgical specialties rotate the day every month so that no one firm will be penalised by loss of outpatient clinics or operating sessions. All consultants and junior staff are requested to attend, and a register is kept. In general surgery the senior registrar organises the audit, and in orthopaedic surgery one consultant and his junior staff are responsible on a rotating basis. This method will be used in the medical specialty, although currently one nominated consultant has arranged each audit meeting. Specialty groups have different approaches to the format of an audit meeting, but an agenda would include a short business meeting, clinical input, and the discussion of an agreed topic. The business item might include discussing problems that affect all the medical staff in that specialty, and topics to be audited at future meetings might be decided. The clinical input might be either a review of mortality or morbidity or a discussion of selected cases of a defined condition or in which lessons might be learnt from the problems that had arisen. The management of a group of cases with a defined diagnosis might be reviewed—for example, subarachnoid haemorrhage or late onset asthma. The last item is usually a topic that may have arisen from peer review, when there is concern or disagreement over clinical management, or it might be about conditions or treatments characterised by high volume or high risk. The purpose is to provide guidelines (or standards) accepted by most of the medical staff as to what constitutes good clinical practice in the diagnosis and management of that particular condition. Standards that have already been defined, evaluated, and published are also used, but they may be adapted for local use or updated when necessary. In the medical unit we use guidelines for medical emergencies and chronic medical conditions published by Bristol and Weston District Health Authority.[1]

In the medical specialties peer review is separate from the main audit meeting and takes place monthly at a lunchtime meeting lasting one hour. Two consultants with their junior staff audit each other, and cases are usually taken at random from the previous four to six weeks' deaths or discharges. This allows discussion of common conditions as distinct from interesting diseases. Peer review is primarily an educational exercise, in which the quality of the notes is freely discussed using a checklist first described by the acute medical unit in Birmingham.[2] We look critically at investigations with special reference to repeat investigations and to those done out of hours. The differential diagnosis often acts as a source for discussion of symptoms and signs, and comments are made on the quality of the follow up notes, with a check to see whether information given to relatives is recorded. The diagnosis on discharge is checked for accuracy, and the discharge summary is checked for content and the date of posting to the general practitioner.

Chesterfield and North Derbyshire Royal Hospital is currently installing a case-mix patient management system, but even within our present resources of two free-standing PCs there has been no difficulty in finding material for audit meetings. We are reviewing the management of everyday problems with a view to recommending guidelines that all consultants in that specialty can accept. For example, the surgeons have now agreed on a common approach to preventing deep vein thrombosis; previously there were three different regimens shared by four consultants. The guidelines for cross matching blood for cold surgery—that is, the amount of blood for each category of operation—have also been accepted.

Many of our meetings are interdisciplinary and include haematologists, anaesthetists, radiologists, and other members of the pathology staff. Each of these groups also has its own meetings.

Problems identified

Quality of medical records—When analysed systematically and critically most records are deficient. During peer review in the medical unit the use of the Birmingham protocol has resulted in considerable improvement over the one year of audit. We also use guidelines from Brighton[3] on what should be in the clinical medical record. A reprint of this article is issued to each member of the junior staff and a copy is kept in a reference file on each ward.

Diagnostic accuracy—The present method of coding diagnosis according to the International Classification of Diseases (ninth revision) is unsatisfactory, although this might be improved shortly by a change to Read coding. We decided that doctors should be responsible for ensuring that the diagnosis recorded in the notes is accurate. This may be decided during a ward round or the junior staff can discuss this with more senior doctors before discharge of the patient. The consultant will be responsible for checking that the diagnostic code is correct. We are debating whether a coding clerk should be allocated to a small group of specialties rather than being responsible for the whole hospital system as at present. Secretaries will become more involved in these procedures and in some specialties may take over the coding. A computer training programme is available for all medical and secretarial staff to illustrate the process of coding.

Retrieving information from notes is extremely difficult without the use of computers. We have collaborated in the design of a flexible clinical information system with Data Med Computer Systems. Pilot trials have been completed, and this system will be introduced gradually to all specialties. Information from resource management will also help.

Small specialties—In specialties with fewer than three consultants interdistrict audit is carried out. Collaboration has been arranged either region wide (for genitourinary medicine and rheumatology) or with four to five adjacent districts (for mental handicap and adolescent psychiatry, ear, nose, and throat and dermatology). Audit of the accident and emergency department still poses the most organisational problems.

Statistical accuracy—Problems have been identified with performance indicators, waiting lists, and outpatient consultations, and the departments of planning and research and medical records have agreed to rectify them.

Outpatient audit poses problems because of the large numbers of patients. Currently being installed is a long awaited computerised database, an outpatient module of the case-mix management system to audit and monitor outpatient activity.

Reproducible measures of outcome and quality of life

In surgery diagnosis, intervention, and outcomes are usually clearly defined. The medical specialties entail multiple interventions, there are various secondary manifestations of disease, and counselling of the patient plays a large part in treatment, and these are difficult measures to define. Currently, we rely on data in textbooks and in published reports (specific articles and clinical trials). Comparison with other districts or with national results is virtually non-existent. Involving patients in measuring outcome is difficult; the questionnaires completed by the patient have limitations, and employing staff to visit patients to help them complete a questionnaire is expensive but would give a more accurate picture.

Liaison with general practitioners about long term outcome has not been established. Telephoning general practitioners at their surgeries—a method used in the United States—would not be popular here, asking them to complete a questionnaire would be time consuming, and limiting the number of questions to try to ensure a reply would limit the value of the results.

The Royal College of Physicians has set up a unit to investigate the problems to try to produce outcomes for common conditions that might be used for national comparison. It has realised for some time that measurement of the quality of life of patients during treatment and thereafter is important. The separation of factors other than treatment that can affect the outcome—for example, age, sex, social circumstances, and depression—will have to be assessed if any meaningful comparisons are to be made.

District medical audit committee

The district audit committee meets monthly and comprises one contact from each specialty and includes the postgraduate tutor, the director of public health, a general practitioner representative, and the audit coordinator and analyst.

In conclusion, the organisation of audit in this district health authority has as one key element the appointment of a senior clinician as coordinator of districtwide audit with adequate administrative back up and information technology support; the other key element is the enthusiastic support of the consultants. Our experience shows that audit can be started without computer technology, but a flexible clinical information system is essential to enhance the process of audit and to extend its scope.

1 Bristol and Weston Health Authority. *The treatment of some medical emergencies and chronic medical conditions*. Bristol: Bristol and Weston Health Authority, 1987.
2 Royal College of Physicians. *Report on medical audit. Form used by the medical unit in Birmingham for regular audit meetings*. London: RCP, 1989:14–5.
3 Bennet J, Shaw CD. Guidance on what should be in the medical records for the Brighton Health District. *Association of Health Care Information and Medical Records Officers Journal* 1987;**28**:103–10.

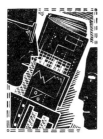

Medical audit data: counting is not enough

CYNTHIA LYONS,
ROBERT GUMPERT

Medical audit is a review of patient care.[1] It necessitates abstracting information from patient records and making judgments about the quality of care given. These judgments are made by considering indicators of structure, process, and outcome.[2,3] Conceptual problems abound, in part because we are dealing with a continuum. It is not clear where structure becomes process and process outcome. An oversimplistic, but nevertheless useful, distinction can be made. Structure audit involves analysing fixed resource inputs; process audit analysing investigations, procedures, and treatments; and outcome audit analysing the assessment of a patient's condition after an episode of treatment.

But what are these indicators of structure, process, and outcome? Can medical audit be used to judge the quality of care given? Several surgical units have reported the development of medical audit,[4-9] but little has been written about the presentation and interpretation of audit data.

Medical audit data are the product of a complicated process. They are a static representation of dynamic processes. In the case of inpatients, for instance, there are many stages between admission and discharge, and medical audit attempts to intercept patients and events at different points along the "process continuum" and make counts. Evaluating these audit data is necessarily a complex exercise. Audit data alone cannot explain: they should be seen only as indicators, not final results. They describe what is there without providing an understanding of the underlying structure.

This paper reports some of the results of the first full year's audit of all inpatients for one consultant general surgeon, drawing particular attention to the problems of interpretation and the need for the careful presentation of data.

Background and method

Since 1985 CASPE Research (clinical accountability, service planning, evaluation) has worked closely with senior clinicians in Brighton on a series of projects funded by the Department of Health research management division to develop measures and information systems for quality assurance. The purpose of the research is to develop indicators of quality, tested by clinicians and other professionals, using self audit.

In September 1985 after careful evaluation of the audit software products on the market,[10] Dunnfile was chosen to help with the routine auditing of consultants' inpatient workload. Dunnfile is a surgical audit software package developed by Mr D C Dunn, a general surgeon in Cambridge. It is used to collect a set of data on every inpatient admission which are used to generate discharge summaries and for surgical audit.

An analysis of all inpatient records relating to one consultant surgeon (RG) for the period 1 January 1988 to 31 December 1988 was undertaken. A total of 859 records were counted. In May 1988 we checked the adequacy of data collection by comparing the numbers of patients on the system with the manual records kept by ward clerks for the three months February to April 1988.

Results and discussion

Procedures

During 1988, 655 main procedures and 79 secondary procedures were performed. (A secondary procedure is performed at the same time as a main procedure.) Knowledge of the number and type of operations performed is interesting in itself, but we also needed information about the surgeon and the complexity of the operation.

By attributing a British United Provident Association (BUPA) code to each main procedure and grouping procedures by the principal surgeon who performed them we produced table I. This shows, for example, that the consultant performed 78% of all

TABLE I—Grades of operation by surgeon: main procedure only

Surgeon	Minor	Intermediate	Major	⩾ Major +	Total
Consultant 1	51	191	74	21	337
Other consultants	0	0	2	1	3
Senior registrar 1	9	12	22	2	45
Senior registrar 2	12	9	14	1	36
Registrar 1	9	27	32	2	70
Registrar 2	4	4	4	0	12
Other senior registrars	0	1	2	0	3
Other registrar	6	9	15	0	30
Senior house officer 1	13	34	4	0	51
Clinical assistant	2	2	0	0	4
Other senior house officers	8	8	13	0	29
House surgeon	0	1	1	0	2
Radiologist	0	13	0	0	13
Anaesthetist	0	0	2	0	2
Other	2	2	2	0	6
Locum registrar	1	8	3	0	12
Total	117	321	190	27	655

operations classified as major+ and above. In addition, and of greater interest in the management of the firm, it shows that registrar 1 performed more major operations than the senior registrars.

Complications

Eighty records (12·2%) noted postoperative complications, nine showing that the patient died. Sixty eight records showed that the patient experienced one complication, and 12 showed two complications. The total number of postoperative complications was therefore 92 (table II). The 80 records represented only 74 admissions, since four patients had two records and one patient had three records. (Dunnfile creates a patient record for each inpatient episode, plus additional records if the patient experiences a return to theatre during a single admission. A patient who experienced two returns to theatre would therefore have three records.)

But simple numerical information about the number and type of complications by itself is not very useful. Further information about the surgeon and the calculation of an overall complication rate made this more meaningful (table III).

TABLE II—Postoperative complications

Complication		No
Death		9
Bleeding problems		14
Wound haemorrhage	1	
Wound haematoma	9	
Gastrointestinal haemorrhage	4	
Infections		34
Chest infection	9	
Wound infection	11	
Wound dehiscence	2	
Urinary infection	3	
Pelvic abscess	1	
Fever (?cause)	5	
Other infection	3	
Thromboembolism		7
Pulmonary embolism	1	
Arterial embolism	1	
Ischaemic leg	4	
Cerebrovascular accident (stroke)	1	
Cardiac problem		5
Myocardial infarction	2	
Other	3	
Urinary problem		6
Retained stone	1	
Retention of urine	3	
Renal failure	2	
Anastomotic problems		3
Leak	2	
Fistula	1	
Other problems		14
Nerve palsy	2	
Confusion	1	
Other*	11	
Total		92

*Other includes: occlusion of graft, chest pain (?cause), pneumothorax, diarrhoea, and persistent vomiting.

Table III shows that registrar 1 had a lower complication rate than the senior registrars, yet, as mentioned earlier (table I), registrar 1 performed more major operations than the senior registrars. It also shows that the anaesthetist had a 100% complication rate, which was misleading, because neither of the complications resulted from the procedure (lumbar sympathetic nerve block). So table III clearly still leaves out important information. The calculation of an overall complication rate does not draw

TABLE III—Complications by surgeon

Surgeon	No of operations	No of records with a complication	Complications as % of operations
Consultant 1	337	42	12·5
Senior registrar 1	45	9	20·0
Senior registrar 2	36	7	19·4
Registrar 1	70	8	11·4
Other senior registrars	3	1	33·3
Other registrar	30	5	16·6
Senior house officer 1	51	3	5·9
Anaesthetist	2	2	100·0
Other	6	2	33·3
Locum registrar	12	1	8·3
Total	592	80	13·5

attention to procedures that are particularly prone to complications for individual surgeons. The analysis of complications, taking into account the complexity of the operation, is more revealing.

Table IV was constructed by calculating a complication rate for each grade of operation the surgeon performed. The percentages are of interest because these could be used to illustrate risk per 100 for each grade of operation. The percentages may also be used to convey the distribution of risk—the relative vulnerability at each grade of operation. For example, for the consultant patients having major + and above operations are at most risk, those having major operations the next most vulnerable, with risk declining with grade of operation, as expected. But why should 25% of intermediate operations by senior registrar 1 result in a complication? Even this complex table does not provide all the answers.

Ultimately, what may be of most interest is whether the complications were avoidable or unavoidable. But such a classification of complications is difficult, even in apparently straightforward cases. For example, the breakdown of an anastomosis between ileum and right colon is theoretically avoidable, although it is a well recognised complication. But who is to say whether or not it is avoidable in a particular case?

Return to theatre

Eighteen (2·2%) patients experienced at least one return to

TABLE IV—Complication by grade of operation by surgeon

	Minor		Intermediate		Major		≥Major+		Total	
	No of complications/ operations	Complication rate (%)	No of complications/ operations	Complication rate (%)	No of complications/ operations	Complication rate (%)	No of complications/ operations	Complication rate (%)	No of complications/ operations	Complication rate (%)
Consultant 1	0/51	0	12/191	6·3	20/74	27·0	10/21	47·6	42/337	12·5
Senior registrar 1	0/9	0	3/12	25·0	5/22	22·8	1/2	50·0	9/45	20·0
Senior registrar 2	0/12	0	2/9	22·2	4/14	28·6	1/1	100	7/36	19·4
Registrar 1	0/9	0	2/27	7·4	6/32	18·8	0/2	0	8/70	11·4
Other senior registrars	0		0/1	0	1/2	50·0	0		1/3	33·3
Other registrar	1/6	16·6	1/9	11·1	3/15	20·0	0		5/30	16·6
Senior house officer 1	0/13	0	3/34	8·9	0/4	0	0		3/51	5·9
Anaesthetist	0		0		2/2	100	0		2/2	100
Other	0/2	0	1/2	50·0	1/2	50	0		2/6	33·3
Locum registrar	0/1	0	1/8	12·5	0/3	0	0		1/12	8·3
Total	1/103	1·0	25/293	8·5	42/170	24·7	12/26	46·0	80/592	13·5

TABLE v — Details of returns to theatre in six patients

Case No	Diagnosis	1st operation	Reason for 2nd operation	2nd operation	Reason for 3rd operation	3rd operation	Reason for 4th operation	4th operation	Other details
1	Femoral embolism	Femoral embolectomy	Insufficient blood supply to leg	Femoral embolectomy + fasciotomy (calf)					Age 66. Stroke 2 weeks before admission. General condition poor. Died
2	Atherosclerosis	Femoral-popliteal bypass graft	Occluded graft	Femoral popliteal distal bypass graft	Occluded graft	Disobliteration of femoral-popliteal graft	Occluded graft	Above knee amputation	Age 71. Smoker
3	Leg embolism	Femoral embolectomy	Insufficient blood supply to leg	Superior femoral artery vein patch + femoral embolectomy					Age 84. History of peripheral vascular disease. Ischaemic heart disease. Poor general condition. Died
4	Colonic carcinoma	Examination under anaesthesia	After initial assessment tumour removal a possibility?	Laparotomy					Age 68. Circumferential tumour around anus, therefore inoperable
5	Atherosclerosis, claudication	Femoral embolectomy	Gastro-intestinal haemorrhage + ischaemic leg	Bleeding duodenal ulcer underrun + vagotomy + pyloroplasty	Insufficient blood supply to leg	Femoral-femoral crossover graft			Age 68. Smoker. Alcoholic. Bleeding duodenal ulcer
6	Leg trauma	Debridement of wound	Insufficient blood supply to leg	Skin graft + debridement of wound	Insufficient blood supply to leg	Debridement of wound			Age 85. Major haematoma. Grafting of necrotic skin

theatre during a single admission. The return to theatre rate cannot be taken as an indicator of poor quality of care without considerable qualification. It is not enough even to consider only unplanned returns to theatre as an indicator. A detailed examination of the patients who experienced a return to theatre is needed. Table V, which examines six patients, is an example of the kind of analysis that is required. Each return to theatre needs to be presented with clinical information which sets it in context.

In the case of vascular surgery multiple returns to theatre during a single admission may occur as a result of occluded grafts (see case 2). The longer a vascular graft is—for example, a femorotibial bypass graft—the more likely it is to thrombose. A vascular surgeon may perform such a graft, knowing that there is a less than 50% chance that the graft will remain patent, because the alternative is a major amputation. So it is not uncommon to perform two or three (or more) operations to try to save a patient's leg but eventually, when all else fails, to amputate it. There is always a chance that the leg could be saved by a particular operation. To amputate straight away would reduce the surgeon's return to theatre rate but would be unethical. Grafts occlude for various reasons, only one of which is technical error. Who is to say, therefore, whether graft occlusion in a particular patient is or is not avoidable? So, as with complications, what may be of most interest is whether the return to theatre was avoidable or unavoidable.

Unplanned returns to theatre are therefore part of the clinical course of some diseases and should not be seen as an indicator of poor quality. The numbers of returns to theatre on their own have little meaning.

Adequacy of data collection

Even though counts alone—of complications, returns to theatre—are not enough, it is important to ensure that the counts are accurate and that data are gathered on all patients. In Brighton the completed data collection forms are sent to a central point for input to the system. But the fact that the consultant's work is spread over three sites and 12 wards makes it difficult to ensure that all inpatient episodes are recorded. When we studied the adequacy of data collection in May 1988 we uncovered a deficit of nearly 30%. We therefore re-examined everyone's role—that is, that of all medical, clerical, and administrative staff—in the whole process. It became clear that day patients, patients admitted to seldom used wards, and patients admitted during the night were being overlooked.

After the completion of the year's audit, we again checked for a shortfall in the numbers of patients entered on to the system. As we were concerned about the accuracy of the ward clerks' manual records we compared our number with the number of patients in the district's patient administration system. We discovered a shortfall of 169 (17%). The audit was carried out five weeks after the end of the year, and some patients, although admitted in 1988, may still have been in hospital. In addition, the absence of staff led to backlogs. Many of the forms would probably eventually have found their way to the computer. But the reasons why some forms never got there were unclear.

Is it worth it?

Three recent publications provide useful explanations of, and guides to, medical audit.[11-13] But it is clear, especially to those who have tried, that systematic medical audit does not come about easily. The use of a computerised audit system includes everyone in a discipline of data collection that is unfamiliar. Protocols have to be set up to ensure that the system works and that data are collected on all inpatients.

Despite our efforts we still have the problem of ensuring a 100% coverage of inpatient workload. Anything less than a 100% coverage considerably devalues the interpretation of audit data. So how, in such circumstances, can audit data be used as a working tool for managing a surgical firm? The timing of audits is only part of the answer, for some inpatient proformas, as already shown, may never get to the computer. If Dunnfile could communicate with the other hospital information systems, such as the patient administrative system, it would be easier and less time consuming to check for and chase up missing or delayed data collection forms. Communication with this system would also reduce the amount of time spent keying in patient information. Demographic details and certain details about the patient's hospital stay already entered into the patient administration system could be down loaded to Dunnfile, eliminating the need to rekey them.

Despite these problems there have been many benefits gained by incorporating routine audits into the day to day running of the surgical firm. The audit has recorded the throughput of the firm and allowed us to show activity objectively.

In general surgery in Brighton, morbidity and mortality meetings have been routine practice since 1984. By recording complications and interesting cases as they occur Dunnfile has made case selection for presentation at such meetings much easier. It has offered us the opportunity to study the incidence and pattern of complications so that any possible improvement or changes in practice can be undertaken. Junior staff are given printouts highlighting the cases they have been concerned with during their training. Information about the number and type of operations and the ensuing complications are readily available. The data generated can be used in managing the firm. A future prospect, requiring more than a year's audit data, could be the tracking of changes in the firm, such as increased specialisation.

Nevertheless, the considerable amount of time and effort that has had to be put in to garner these benefits should not be understated. The quality of the data depends on the commitment and enthusiasm of the whole firm, but in particular the consultant. The actual process of filling in forms for audit has significantly changed clinical practice. A data collection form has to be filled in for all inpatients; the surgeon performing an operation is responsible for filling in the appropriate details, and all the information on the data collection forms is then verified by the consultant before being entered on to the computer.

Consideration has to be given to the mode of presentation of audit data. Dunnfile produced most of the information we demanded of it. But only in a few cases could the information be incorporated into other reports without further work. Some tabulations had to be done manually—for example, that showing complications by grade of operation by surgeon (table IV). Other information, we decided, could be more appropriately presented in graph form.

Time spent considering the presentation of data, so that it can make apparent aspects and regularities which might otherwise be difficult to discern, is time well spent. Unless great care is taken over the presentation of audit data (and even when data presentation has been meticulous) the data are open to misuse:

The secret language of statistics, so appealing in a fact minded culture, is employed to sensationalise, inflate, confuse and oversimplify. Statistical methods and statistical terms are necessary in reporting the mass data of social and economic trends, business conditions, "opinion polls," the census. But without writers who use the words with honesty and understanding and readers who know what they mean the result can only be semantic nonsense.[14]

What we have attempted to do in this paper is to raise awareness about the problems of presenting and interpreting audit data and to illustrate this by questioning the appropriateness of using such generally accepted (but crude) indicators of quality such as the numbers of complications and returns to theatre without further qualification.

1 Department of Health. *NHS review working paper 6. Medical audit.* London: DoH:3.
2 Donabedian A. Evaluating the quality of medical care. *Millbank Memorial Fund Quarterly* 1966;**44**:166–206.
3 Donabedian A. *Explorations in quality assessment and monitoring.* Vol 1. *The definition of quality and approaches to its assessment.* Ann Arbor, Michigan: Health Administration Press, 1980.
4 Stock S, Young M, Hardiman P, Petty A. A microcomputer based system for surgical audit. *British Journal of Clinical Practice* 1985;July:261–6.
5 Campbell W, Souter R, Collin J, Wood R, Kidson I, Morris P. Auditing the vascular surgical audit. *Br J Surg* 1987;**74**:98–100.
6 Ellis B, Michie H, Esufali S, Pyper R, Dudley H. Development of a microcomputer-based system for surgical audit and patient administration: a review. *J R Soc Med* 1987; **80**:157–61.
7 Dunn D. Audit of a surgical firm by microcomputer: five years' experience. *Br Med J* 1988;**296**:687–91.
8 Glass R, Thomas P. Surgical audit in a district general hospital: a stimulus for improving patient care. *Ann R Coll Surg Engl* 1987;**69**:135–9.
9 Gumpert R. Why on earth do surgeons need quality assurance? *Ann R Coll Surg Engl* 1988;**70**:261.
10 Stevens G. Selecting computer software packages—a self-help guide: discussion paper. *J R Soc Med* 1988;**81**:458–60.
11 Shaw C. *Medical audit: a handbook.* London: King's Fund Centre, 1989.
12 Royal College of Physicians. *Medical audit; a first report: what, why and how?* London: RCP, 1989.
13 Royal College of Surgeons of England. *Guidelines to clinical audit in surgical practice.* London: RCS, 1989.
14 Huff D. *How to lie with statistics.* London: Victor Gollancz, 1954.

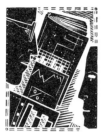

A clinician's guide to setting up audit

BRIAN W ELLIS, TOM SENSKY

By April 1991 the Department of Health expects medical audit to be implemented in every hospital. The implementation of some district audit programmes has already been described.[1][2] In Hounslow and Spelthorne the district audit advisory committee was concerned with the need to disseminate an understanding of audit, dispel a fear of the process, and provide sufficient guidance to enable clinicians to implement audit. To that end it produced a guide of its plans and the necessary actions, which was sent to every consultant in the district. (The districts have two general hospitals: Ashford and West Middlesex University Hospitals.) A covering letter requested the consultants to complete a confidential questionnaire designed to help identify current strengths and deficiencies in audit, which is essential in planning how to share expertise and resources throughout the district. Within three weeks completed questionnaires had been received from more than 60% of the recipients. This paper is a synopsis of the circulated document.

How to set up audit

Intended for guidance rather than as a rulebook, the document had three principal aims.

- To review the background and basic principles of clinical audit.
- To illustrate some of the methods of audit.
- To give general guidance on implementing audit.

Background and basic principles

What is clinical audit?—The Department of Health defines audit as: "The systematic, critical analysis of the quality of medical care, including the procedures used for diagnosis and treatment, the use of resources, and the resulting outcome and quality of life for the patient," and states that "an effective programme of medical audit will help to provide reassurance to doctors, their patients, and managers that the best quality of service is being achieved, *having regard to the resources available.*"[3] Clinical audit and resource management have much in common. The data required for both overlap considerably and the information derived in each is relevant to the other.[4] However, clinical audit is the responsibility of clinicians and must be led by them.[5] The district committee views audit as safeguarding the clinical care of patients against inappropriate change dictated by economy.

Educational value of audit*

- Critical review of current practice and comparisons against predefined standards encourages acquisition and updating of knowledge
- Identification of key features of clinical practice allows relevant lessons to be learnt
- Through audit, it is possible to identify particular areas where knowledge could be improved or is deficient, suggesting the need for research
- Self evaluation and peer review are important components of postgraduate education

*Standing Committee on Postgraduate Medical Education[5]

Educational aspects—The educational benefits of clinical audit (box) have been considered in depth by Batstone.[6] The committee believes that reviewing the lessons arising from previous audit meetings and ensuring that the conclusions of those meetings have been acted on is fundamentally important.[7] Some departments have found it necessary to devote a whole meeting every six to 12 months to this purpose alone; it is essential that the educational potential of clinical audit is realised.

Responsibilities for clinical audit—Regional health authorities are responsible for ensuring that all doctors are participating in medical audit by April 1991: they will also facilitate cooperative audit between hospital and community authorities and coordinate global audit (see below), which entails collecting regional data, setting regional standards, and comparing against these the practice of individual units or clinicians. Our regional health authority has accepted the district medical audit implementation plan (box) produced by the district committee, which is now being implemented.

District medical audit implementation plan

- A strategy and timetable for developing audit
- Organisation of audit and a description of types of audit to be used
- Requirements for information and information technology
- Staffing requirements (audit coordinator and assistants)
- Training and educational strategies
- Policy on confidentiality
- Identification of a budget holder
- Explicit mechanisms for regular reporting of audit results to management

---

District audit advisory committee—Within the district this committee will supervise audit. Four clinicians representing a range of clinical and service specialties from each of the acute units and representatives from the community health unit and from management will make up the committee. They will be helped by an audit coordinator. The committee will report to the district medical advisory committee.

Unit audit committee—The four district committee representatives from each unit will themselves form the unit audit committee, together with the clinical tutor, a senior nurse, and a local general practitioner. Their objectives are broadly similar to those of the district audit advisory committee (box). In addition they include:

- Communicating between firms or groups of doctors and the advisory committee, each clinical representative being responsible for several departments or clinical specialties
- Identifying a lead clinician within each specialty and through him or her encouraging audit for every doctor in the unit and receiving the results of audit
- Liaising with and directing audit assistants locally
- Liaising with their medical staff committees.

Planning audit in your unit—The person responsible for audit in a department will need to consider:

- Who should be involved in the audit process
- What method(s) of audit to use
- How and by whom data will be collected
- How often to meet and for how long
- What to do with the results
- The educational aspects
- What resources will be needed
- How to preserve confidentiality.

A complete system of audit should not be attempted in a single step; it would be an advantage to plan several stages in the development of the audit process starting, for example, with case note review. The evolution of the process will require regular monitoring.

Who should participate?—All doctors must participate, but for audit to succeed *a clear commitment to it is required by senior medical staff*. In most specialties audit will be done independently at each hospital, but in specialties in which the number of consultants are small, joint input from staff at both district hospitals would be better. Involving health care professionals other than doctors in audit is considered valuable to the audit process and to the improvement of education and communication.[58] Most specialties require interdisciplinary collaboration, and a fundamental principle of audit should be to encourage the development of multidisciplinary audit procedures. Thus surgeons should meet with anaesthetists and psychiatrists with social workers, etc. Because of their close working relation nurses should be closely involved in most aspects of audit; they should also consider independently how to audit their care. A good case can be made for involving clinicians in the same specialty from another hospital, which should permit a different perspective on clinical problems—with potential educational and clinical benefits. Regular participation, however, is probably impracticable. Because the chief aim of audit is to improve the service for patients, their participation also needs to be considered[9]; this is a longer term aim, to be used under clearly defined circumstances.

Methods of audit

The district committee classified audit activities as follows in order to have a clear definition of terms. The first two categories are the essential audit activities of any department offering clinical services; the third (case note review) is considered mandatory for any department offering continuing inpatient care. The committee intends to review the proposed audit plans for each specialty to formulate agreed schemes, from which will emerge the degree of support required from audit assistants and the structure of reporting. We hope that some departments will bid for the use of audit assistants for well defined projects.

Objectives of the district audit advisory committee

- Coordinate and foster clinical audit for every doctor in the district
- Determine existing audit practice in all clinical departments
- Assist clinicians in all departments in implementing audit methods (see text)
- Monitor results and conclusions of the audit process
- Monitor validity of data and reporting
- Encourage more elaborate forms of audit, when appropriate
- Ensure that changes, when indicated by the outcome of audit, are implemented
- Ensure that audit is an integral part of education
  - —That the outcome of audit is perceived as educational
  - —That doctors are educated in the practice and process of audit
- Endeavour to minimise the perception that audit is threatening and to highlight the benefits of the audit process to doctors and patients
- Train and direct audit assistants
- Ensure effective liaison with
  - —district medical advisory committee
  - —management
  - —general practitioners
  - —the community unit
- Maintain confidentiality
- Estimate funding required for audit
- Prepare annual report
- Prepare forward programme

For a further perspective on the role of a district audit committee see Gumpert and Lyons[2]

Basic clinical audit entails an analysis of throughput and a broad analysis of case type, complications, and morbidity and mortality.

Such data should be reviewed by each clinical firm at intervals of about three months. When possible, the results should be contrasted with previous periods of time, other clinical firms, other hospitals, or information derived from global audit (see below).

Incident review entails discussing strategies for clinical scenarios. An incident may be taken to be anything from a patient having a cardiac arrest to the use of a department for an investigation—for example, emergency intravenous urography. Such discussions are expected to lead to clear policies. This method is particularly suitable for multidisciplinary or interdisciplinary audit.

Clinical record review—A clinical firm invites a member of another firm of the same or similar specialty to review a random selection of case notes, against established criteria when possible. Such audit has the advantage of simplicity and requires little additional time or other resources. A potential disadvantage, however, is too much concentration on the quality of record keeping and not enough on patient care—both of which are distinct, though related facets of the clinical process. In practice, a balance between the two might be encouraged by the audit meetings being chaired by a third clinician who is neither auditing nor being audited.

Criterion audit is a more advanced and structured form of incident audit. Various incidents are analysed retrospectively against several carefully chosen criteria, which should encapsulate the key elements in management and be discernible from the medical record by a non-medical audit assistant. All cases falling within the scope of the topic are screened, and those failing to meet any one of the criteria are selected for further clinical review. The criteria may relate to administrative elements (for example, waiting time), investigations, treatments considered, outcome, follow up strategies, etc. This form of audit entails much preliminary discussion and research by audit assistants. Experience suggests that it is usually worthwhile.[10]

Screening of adverse occurrences—A clinical firm decides on a shortlist of events that should be avoided—for example, wound infections, bedsores, suicides, etc. The frequency and factors leading up to each case at the occurrence of these events is analysed.[11]

Focused audit studies—The outcome of any audit may require a more closely focused area of research, which is similar to an academic research exercise.

Global audit—Commonly, in any hospital few departments perform similar work. The case mix even between the mainstream physicians or surgeons may be sufficiently different to negate the value of a comparative audit. In other specialties there may not be others in the hospital with whom to compare results. Global audit implies collecting and comparing data across units, districts, and even throughout a region.[12 13] Surgeons in this district already contribute data to the regional surgical audit global audit programme; the obstetricians and gynaecologists participate in global audit of obstetric and perinatal data; and four accident and emergency departments (including both at our acute units) are active in global audit. The committee's view is that global audit should be encouraged, particularly among smaller specialties.

Audit of outcome is probably the most difficult, controversial, and time consuming exercise. Generally, outcome will probably depend on the whole process of health care delivery during an episode of a patient's treatment in hospital and as such is a measure of the range of skills of the medical and nursing staff, the administration, and, indeed, every person or department the patient has contact with. More simply, aspects of outcome may be measured by a criterion audit approach. The committee will propose studies to assess the contrast between the perspectives on outcome between the patient, the general practitioner, and the clinician and also to measure the patient's perspective on outcome at the end of hospital admission and several months later.

Patients and communications—As audit is concerned with improving the service to patients the committee will develop techniques to test service provision from the patients' perspective. There will be emphasis on ensuring good communication between doctors, all health care professionals, and especially their patients.

Many of these audit methods will be applied generally; investigations will also be targeted on treatments or conditions that are either common or associated with high morbidity, high mortality, or long stay. Many departments are actively implementing audit; some have been running audit for many years, and in some specialties audit is an absolute requirement for accreditation for higher training.

Implementing audit

The time required for audit will be appreciable for all concerned. Clinicians responsible for particular elements of audit work will require even more time, but such responsibility should rotate. The frequency of audit meetings will depend on the type of audit being performed; a monthly meeting of about 60–90 minutes is recommended as a minimum. *It is important that the clinician charged with organising audit within the specialty produces a clear plan and timetable so that all doctors in the specialty know precisely what is expected of them.* Firms that run clinical information systems may need internal weekly meetings to discuss the previous week's discharges and validate their data entry; such meetings are important but are no substitute for a structured audit meeting.

Reporting results—Detailed minutes of audit meetings are not appropriate, but the nature and outcome of every audit must be recorded.[10] The person responsible for audit within a department must agree with his or her colleagues who is responsible for documentation; this may be whoever is chairing the meeting. A report must be prepared and marked as confidential. It should be kept by the person with lead responsibility for audit in the unit and a copy sent to the district committee representative for the specialty. If audit results are considered relevant to another service or professional group you may determine how the information is to be shared.

Staffing—Initially, it is important to plan audit activity that can be realistically achieved with existing staff. More elaborate forms of audit may require the help of audit assistants, and implementing computerised audit systems entails much effort in collecting and validating data to achieve complete data capture.[14] Clinical and non-clinical staff in each department will need to participate in audit, and part of their time will need to be so allocated. This commitment must be recognised in resources and funding. An audit coordinator and two audit assistants have been appointed, and the district committee hopes that departments will submit protocols for audit involving these assistants. By contrast, the committee may approach departments with proposals for district-wide projects with help from audit assistants.

Clinical information systems—Specialties already running computerised information systems will have rapid access to data analysed in a fashion suitable for audit.[15] Some regional funding will be used to help more firms install such systems. Clinical audit, however, is not entirely dependent on computers and computerised databases; implementing those audit methods not dependent on computers—audit involving patients' records, some form of incident audit, etc—should not be delayed.

Confidentiality—Information about patients used in audit must protect their confidentiality and that of the professionals. The district committee has drafted guidelines on confidentiality. A consistent policy on confidentiality across the district is vital, particularly when audit activities cross boundaries between specialties or professional disciplines. The same principles are involved in patient confidentiality as in the clinical conferences that form part of any academic programme. The matter becomes more complex if professionals other than doctors are involved in audit. It will be important to secure a commitment from all those concerned not to discuss the content of an audit meeting elsewhere. Unless an explicit and convincing case can be made for including details that identify a patient in verbal or written presentations, they should be excluded. Protecting the confidentiality of the professionals will probably prove difficult in some types of audit—for example, when one consultant reviews the clinical records of another consultant's patient or when reviewing patients who have been in hospital longer than three months. Nevertheless, this type of audit can be successful, provided that the necessary atmosphere of trust and collaboration is fostered. Some types of audit are more likely to precipitate interpersonal conflict than others. What should happen if audit discloses problems or deficiencies in an individual doctor's practice? The person performing the audit is responsible for feedback to the individual clinician and to the person to whom he or she is professionally responsible (for example, the consultant in the case of junior staff). Only when evidence exists of persistent problems or deficiencies in practice, despite such feedback, should others such as the district committee become involved. In the case of consultants the committee must consider what action should be suggested. The district committee's representative will be able to let you see the guidelines on confidentiality.

1 McConnachie RW. Organisation of audit in North Derbyshire District Health Authority. *BMJ* 1990;**300**:1566–8.
2 Gumpert R, Lyons C. Setting up a district audit programme. *BMJ* 1990;**301**:162–5.
3 Secretaries of State for Health, Wales, Northern Ireland, and Scotland. *Medical audit. Working paper 6*. London: HMSO, 1989.
4 Ellis BW, Rivett RC, Dudley HAF. Extending the use of clinical audit data: a resource planning model. *BMJ* 1990;**301**:159–62.
5 Standing Committee on Postgraduate Medical Education. *Medical audit: the educational implications*. London: SCOPME, 1989.
6 Batstone GF. Educational aspects of medical audit. *BMJ* 1990;**301**:326–8.
7 Smith T. Medical audit. *BMJ* 1990;**300**:65.
8 Nixon SJ. Defining essential hospital data. *BMJ* 1990;**300**:380–1.

9 Anderson J. Patient power in mental health. *BMJ* 1989;**299**:1477–8.
10 Shaw CD, Costain DW. Guidelines for medical audit: seven principles. *BMJ* 1989;**299**:498–9.
11 Bennet J, Walshe K. Occurrence screening as a method of audit. *BMJ* 1990;**300**:1248–51.
12 Ellis BW. Clinical audit. *Br J Hosp Med* 1988;**39**:187.
13 Gruer R, Gordon DS, Gunn AA, Ruckley CV. Audit of surgical audit. *Lancet* 1986;i:23–6.
14 Lyons C, Gumpert R. Medical audit data: counting is not enough. *BMJ* 1990;**300**:1563–6.
15 Ellis BW. How to set up an audit. *BMJ* 1989;**298**:1635–7.

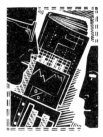

Impact of medical audit advisory groups

CLIVE RICHARDS

Medical audit is a key feature of recent changes to the NHS and is an essential part of the new contract for general practice. Although the term medical audit is used freely, it is necessary to define it. Many definitions have been attempted, but all have in common a systematic critical analysis of aspects of quality of care, reference to standards of care, and commitment to change. Medical audit is not a synonym for traditional review or research activities, as emphasised recently in the report *The Quality of Medical Care*[1] by the government's standing medical advisory committee in its robust statement that "the essential nature of medical audit is a frank discussion between doctors, on a regular basis and without fear of criticism, of the quality of care provided as judged against agreed standards but in a context which allows evolutionary change in such standards."

Medical audit for family doctors is complicated by additional audits of their contractual obligations—for example, measurement of procedures for payment. Audit activities must differentiate between contractual audit, which is a management task whose prime purpose is control, and medical audit, which is a professional task with a prime purpose of education. The dividing line between these two types of audit is often blurred, and the skills and resources for each can be shared. Often the crucial difference between the two will be that of intention. An audit of prescribing to exert downward pressure on costs is clearly a contractual audit and a managerial activity whereas the same procedure undertaken voluntarily to develop a logical treatment policy is a medical audit and an educational activity. Any organised medical audit activity in general practice must acknowledge this distinction.

Structure

The formal mechanism for organising medical audit in general practice will be via a new committee, the medical audit advisory group, structural arrangements for which were described in *Medical Audit in the Family Practitioner Services* health circular (HC (FP)(90) 8). The group will be a committee of the family health services authority, which will appoint its members. There will be up to 12 medically qualified members, most of whom will be general practitioner principals appointed after consultation to ensure that they command the confidence of the profession locally. Appointment to the group will take into account factors such as the distribution of urban and rural practices and the sex and ethnic composition of the local general practitioners. In addition, the group will contain doctors with recognised skill and experience of medical audit. The circular also suggests appointment of a local consultant associated with audit activities in the hospital services and a public health physician. The group will also need to liaise with those responsible for postgraduate medical education, and so the general practitioner members will need to include representatives of the important local and regional educational organisations.

The group will elect its own chairperson and will be responsible to the family health services authority for:

- Ensuring that all practitioners take part in regular and systematic medical audit
- Establishing adequate procedures to protect confidentiality
- Establishing mechanisms to tackle problems disclosed by audit
- Providing a report on the general results of the audit programme.

The circular required that all groups should be established by April 1991 and should institute regular and systematic audit involving all practitioners by April 1992.

Process

The ways in which the groups will work will depend on the philosophy underlying the profession's approach to quality of care. The traditional way has been to identify practices that vary from the norm and eliminate poor performance. It is this model that seems to have inspired some of the thinking behind the proposed establishment of visiting audit teams outlined in the health circular. For many years doctors from the Regional Medical Service visited practices to find out about high prescribing. An alternative is based on theories of continuous improvement, in which good performers are invited to pursue better ways of doing what they already do well. Medical audit should be as much concerned with sharing, publishing, and teaching good examples of care as with exposing bad care. Numerous examples exist of this system in action.[2] In the United States, with its already considerable experience of quality assurance, the Institute of Medicine of the National Academy of Sciences has just released a report on quality assurance for the Medicare Program, which has changed its emphasis from utilisation and cost control to an orientation towards continuous improvement in care.[3]

The management philosophy of the family health services authority will affect the relationship of the medical audit advisory group to individual practices. Many authorities are considering audit networks based on devolution to local units. It is impracticable for a single medical audit advisory group to carry out audit in an authority that may contain over 300 general practitioners, and it will need to set up local advisory groups. The recommendations of the standing medical advisory committee for appointing a local medical audit coordinator[1] may be best effected at a level below that of the authority. Only the smallest authorities will be able to stick to the initial outline in the Department of Health's circular and utilise key members of the medical audit advisory group to work with groups of practices.

All medical audit advisory groups will face common problems.

Meetings—The groups must have a suitable location for meeting and must meet regularly. Apart from work in their own practices, members of the group will have other audit responsibilities, including practice visiting. Active members of the group may have difficulty in meeting their other obligations under the "26 hours over five days" rule for availability in practice. The standing committee's recommendations that a local medical audit coordinator should have four to five sessions per week will be impossible for full time general practitioners, and efforts should be directed to devising alternative solutions.

Resources—Audit has considerable implications for resources. Estimates from the four pilot family health services authorities that have been pioneering medical audit suggest that £100 000 per year is the likely sum required to provide the infrastructure for audit. Failure of the Department of Health to identify and ring fence money for medical audit in primary care, in contrast with its specific allocation of £30m for audit in the hospital and community services, has meant that most family health services authorities are having to set up medical audit as one of many competing priorities for limited funds. None the less, unless medical audit advisory groups are properly resourced at their inception, audit is likely to remain a peripheral activity. The quality of medical audit achieved will reflect the time available to doctors and depend on the number, calibre, and training of support staff. Audit may eventually identify procedures that are wasteful and release resources for other purposes, but this will be a long term benefit.

Examples of audit activities for general practice

Practice activity analysis—Collecting data prospectively and then pooling and analysing them to compare individual performances

Case analysis—Retrospective examination of management in a sample of cases

Disease audit—Assessment of performance for disease management against agreed criteria

Consumer surveys—Using patients' views about aspects of care

Use of routinely available information—Analysis of routine data such as the recently developed service indicators for family health services authorities

Practice annual reports—Their use for audit has been limited, but their future role is likely to be extensive

Critical incident analysis—Regular reviews of selected activities in which an error can be shown to have occurred, such as a complaint from a patient, a visit not logged, or a prescription not issued

---

Confidentiality—Problems of confidentiality in medical audit have yet to be fully dealt with. The main difference between patients' records and audit information is that records are about individual patients whereas audit information is about doctors and is often produced in a form that compares doctors with one another. The degree to which this information should be available to the public has not been agreed. In view of the lack of any privilege relating to its subsequent use in legal proceedings, some doctors are recommending that all information retained by medical audit advisory groups be stripped of identifying detail and limited to basic information such as dates, names of doctors attending meetings, topics discussed, and recommendations in general; all other audit papers should be destroyed. Doctors taking part in audit activities should be bound to hold the proceedings in strict medical confidence. Any report that the group makes will have to be phrased in general terms so that no practice or doctor can be identified. There is therefore a difficult tension between the requirements for keeping information confidential and those for looking at identified problems.

Participation—Ensuring the participation of all doctors will not be easy. Although audit is not yet a part of the terms and conditions of service, there is little doubt that the regulations will be changed if appreciable numbers of doctors do not participate.

Outcome

Many groups will start work with a descriptive survey of audit activities already taking place, thus providing initial suggestions for good practice and identifying topics of local interest and concern. The survey will also describe the degree of variation in local practice and may suggest a direction for future activities. The group may try to institute one type of audit across the whole district—for example, an audit of the management of a chronic disease—or it may adopt an audit policy for each individual practice. District audit is likely to be favoured by managers, who will be keen to show specific activities in return for the resources provided. On the other hand, practices are much more likely to become involved in auditing topics in which they are interested or concerned.[4] Many possibilities for audit activities exist and these have been well described.[5][6] The box shows some examples.

The medical audit advisory group will need to report its activities, and these requirements are outlined in the health circular. A report to the family health services authority will be mandatory and will have to be composed with respect for confidentiality. In addition, the group may also inform other bodies with an interest in its findings, including those responsible for service provision and postgraduate education.

In summary, medical audit advisory groups are a new tool for improving medical care, which will need to be introduced with caution. As with all new medical activities, initial benefits in the hands of enthusiasts may be tempered by the subsequent onset of side effects when the activity is more widely applied. There are many concerns about audit, and the groups will need to ensure that audit activities can show effectiveness. Participation in audit is not necessarily the same as achieving change. As with any form of audit, the group will need to monitor its own performance. It is inevitable, too, that from time to time audit activities will fail, and the group will need to be able to assess these failures and give constructive advice. It should also be willing to disseminate ideas about good practice and to provide suggestions for improvements based on local experience. If handled carefully the impact of medical audit advisory groups will be a beneficial influence on the direction of general practice in the next decade.

1 Department of Health. *The quality of medical care, report of the standing medical advisory committee for the secretaries of state for health and Wales.* London: HMSO, 1990.
2 Irvine DH. *Managing for quality in general practice. Medical audit series 2.* London: King's Fund, 1990.
3 Lohr KN, Schroeder SA. A strategy for quality assurance in Medicare. *N Engl J Med* 1990;**322**:707–12.
4 Baker R, Presley P. *The practice audit plan. A handbook of medical audit for primary health care teams.* Bristol: Royal College of General Practitioners, Severn Faculty, 1990.
5 Hughes J, Humphrey C. *Medical audit in general practice. A practical guide to the literature. Medical audit series 3.* London: King's Fund, 1990.
6 Marinker M (ed). *Medical audit and general practice.* London: BMJ, 1990.

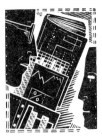

The role of the audit analyst

CHRISTINA FIELDING

In February 1990 I was appointed to a post subsequently entitled audit analyst within the clinical audit department in North Derbyshire Health Authority. With no previous experience in NHS administration I found preparing for the interview difficult. The short job description had mentioned responsibility for data collection and input in two specific projects—in anaesthetics and psychiatry; further information was difficult to locate.

My previous training included nursing and information technology, the second proving to be the most valuable for audit work. I came to realise that the most apt part of the job description was the statement: "... and any other duties appropriate to the position." This reflected the early stages of people's understanding of audit. There are no precedents in this job, and initiative is important; already, methods adopted in February are being changed and updated.

The consultant audit coordinator, Dr McConnachie, had been involved in developing audit in North Derbyshire since 1987. By the time I was appointed funding had been arranged and consultants were showing interest and expressing a need for help with projects. At that time we worked for the district and there were possibilities for audit in many different hospitals. Now a separate community audit team has been formed, and we have been devolved to unit level.

An audit secretary was appointed soon after me and our first days were spent training in the medical records department. The aim was to ease the workload of that department and of the medical secretaries. We now collect all patients' notes ourselves, and any doctor who asks the medical records department for notes for audit is referred to us. The secretary attends the audit meetings for most specialties, takes minutes, collates figures, and distributes agendas, thereby ensuring that this extra work does not fall on the medical secretaries.

Working practice

Since February the clinical audit team, comprising the consultant audit coordinator, the secretary, and myself, has developed a system for audit (figure). The coordinator reads relevant articles and presents his ideas at meetings with consultants in each specialty. He stimulates, motivates, and supervises audit in all specialty groups in the acute unit, paying special attention to those not already active in audit. He sends photocopies of particularly interesting articles to the relevant specialties with comments suggesting possible improvements in practice. Some consultants are enthusiastic but have much to learn about the purpose of the clinical audit team and how it can work for them; many have been collecting and storing information for years, and we are now analysing some of this retrospectively. If the team expands we hope to implement our own ideas for audit studies, but presently we respond to consultants' requests for help with particular projects and have a rapidly increasing workload.

When an idea for audit has been identified by a consultant or

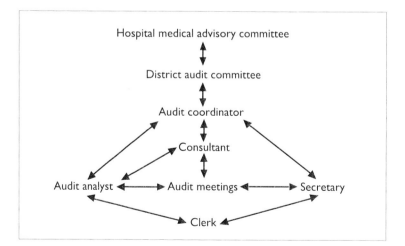

Working of clinical audit team

specialty the consultant(s) and the analyst meet to work out a method of conducting the audit. The objective and the desired improvements are discussed and questions identified for extracting appropriate information. The consultant first describes the present treatment—methods, alternatives, advantages, and disadvantages—to provide background knowledge for the study. For the audit analyst unfamiliarity with medical terms is a hurdle to overcome. With thorough research before starting the study it need not affect the outcome, and this is one of the most satisfying aspects of the job.

Setting up a project

The methotrexate study

An initial meeting was held with a new consultant who wished to obtain more information about patients attending the psoriasis clinic, specifically those being treated with methotrexate, a potentially dangerous drug that requires careful monitoring. He requested an update on their treatment so far, and he had itemised each piece of information he needed to be extracted from the notes (an unusual but extremely helpful step).

After initial discussion about the drug and its effects I asked some fairly standard questions.

(1) What are the alternatives?
(2) How often is the drug administered?
(3) What is an average dose and the outside limits prescribed?
(4) How many patients are receiving this treatment—Do you have a list of them or where can I get one from?
(5) How big is the sample to be used? (In this case it included all of the patients, amounting to 73.)
(6) In which section of the notes may each piece of information be found?

I always seek explanations of any possible abbreviations that may be used in notes. They are often so familiar to the medical staff that they don't mention them, but being unaware of their meaning or ignoring them can lead to inaccuracy in the results.

After the meeting a form was drawn up, incorporating all the information required that could be put on to a database and the form was later retained by the consultant as a record. At this stage a pilot study with about five sets of notes was performed to check that the information on the form could be retrieved. Once the consultant had checked the suitability of the form a database record format was created. The form and the database are often altered and updated during the study as information collected alters the recording requirements of a project.

Current workload

At any one time there are between five and 15 projects underway. More and more frequently, the completed results from projects are required for a certain date—for an audit meeting or a presentation—thereby placing increasing pressure on the analyst/project worker to prioritise the workload thoughtfully.

For most studies the patient's notes are used to look at past treatment or a form to monitor current treatment is created for the medical staff to complete as they see each patient. The information from the completed forms is entered on to a database, either in the audit offices or in the specialty department concerned, depending on who wants to analyse the information. In some cases, such as in the outpatient glaucoma clinic, the forms are used within the department to update and edit the information on the database after each outpatient visit; current details on each patient are then always available for reference by consultants. In others the forms are collected by the audit staff and the information is analysed quarterly, six monthly, or yearly and presented in report and graph form for discussion at audit meetings. The data are analysed but not interpreted. Any obvious improvements are discussed by the audit coordinator and the consultant concerned. The coordinator sees all reports before they are distributed. The audit department has recently started evaluating improvements made six months after the project has finished, thereby recording progress and ensuring that our own work is worthwhile.

Some audit meetings are attended by the audit analyst (with consultants' permission), sufficient to maintain an update of progress within a specialty. Information from meetings not attended may be obtained from the audit secretary or from the minutes of the meetings. The meetings are an excellent way of meeting the medical staff and discussing their views on audit and the methods they prefer to use. All specialties now hold regular meetings but their content varies tremendously—from peer review to general management and the role of the clinical director within audit.

Experience in creating databases to suit various needs is essential to the audit analyst, and the ability to use a word processor is particularly useful. Possible areas in which more training would be appreciated include design of computerised forms, advanced graphics, and statistical analysis.

Projects that involve the clinical audit team include:

- A computerised audit of anaesthetics in all operations performed
- A study of admissions and discharges in psychiatry
- Three studies for the genitourinary clinic, relating to genital warts, their treatment, and relation with cervical cancer in women, and a project determining incidence of chlamydia in cases of termination of pregnancy and the incidence of testing
- Helping the haematology department to create a database of diagnoses in all outpatients and a study of the relation between anticoagulation and atrial fibrillation
- Analysis of records of all patients kept by the orthodontic department since 1984 according to waiting time, diagnosis, type and length of treatment, rate of non-attendance, and outcome
- Analysis of the treatment and outcome of all major trauma patients over the past year
- An audit of the activity in the observation ward
- A study of the use of methotrexate treatment in patients with psoriasis and review of investigations in patients with leg ulcers
- Standardisation of patient care in the coronary care unit by checking procedures relating to diagnosis for all patients in one month and repeating the process during the same month next year. Improvement of information given on echocardiograms to create more meaningful reports
- A study of all resuscitation attempts, their outcome, times of occurrence, and attendance and training of staff
- A quarterly report of epidurals showing the total number of epidurals, the time of day performed, the grade of doctor, the indication, and any complications
- An ongoing database study for the glaucoma clinic to monitor deterioration of vision and effectiveness of treatment.

In other projects help is provided merely by obtaining patients' notes, so clerical help is essential to cover this and other time consuming duties—for example, photocopying—to facilitate the work of the audit team.

Many districts, including North Derbyshire, are in the process of installing case-mix information systems which, although providing valuable information for audit, will also require the development of computer skills within audit departments.

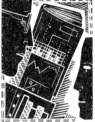

Audit officers: what are they up to?

JENNY FIRTH-COZENS, PAMELA VENNING

Audit assistants, audit officers or coordinators, research officers, facilitators—it seems that the range of titles of those people whose task should be purely audit is bettered only by the large differences in their job descriptions and the actual activity they find themselves undertaking. This article outlines some of the variety of their backgrounds and experiences in their new roles, roles which some see as crucial to the success of the medical audit programme.

Where do audit officers come from?

It is fascinating to witness, emerging from such a diversity of backgrounds, a new professional group in which there is already enough feeling of cohesion to encourage it to form its own professional society. Audit officers have come together from several occupations within the NHS—psychology, medical records, nursing, secretarial, physiotherapy, laboratory, and information services—and from some areas outside the health service, such as computing, commerce, and academia. Their backgrounds seem perhaps less important than their ability to adapt and to think logically, to deal tactfully and helpfully with groups of consultants, to enjoy data and their analysis and presentation, and to get things done. Some people do feel, however, that at least some previous steeping in NHS culture is useful, especially if it has provided a knowledge of clinical terms.

Role and rewards

Our experience is that a good audit officer can and should take part in every stage of the audit cycle. Officers should be present at the design so that they can facilitate discussion on the question being asked and on the purpose of the audit and point out (more usefully for being non-clinicians) the need for precision in definitions and standards: "How will I, as a non-clinician, know that this has been achieved?" is a vital question if data are to be in any way objective. They should agree how data will be collected—by themselves or by a clerk or other professional—and they should analyse the data and present the results back to the specialty group. If officers find some aspects of these activities difficult then these should be addressed in training: the extra funding provided for establishing audit this year cannot be better spent than in providing training for a group that has been, in some places, expected to metamorphose into experts overnight.

This is the average role, the post most commonly called audit officer or coordinator, for which the salary is around £14 000 on scale 5. Below these posts are those of audit clerks, who are often on scale 3, who enter and perhaps collect data and provide the simplest of analyses. Above audit officers or coordinators are rarer individuals, usually called audit facilitators: those who coordinate audit activity across the district, who are on senior management salaries of £18 000 and above. There are still large anomalies in job descriptions and the salaries that accompany them, and it will be a task of the newly formed society to try to reduce such variation.

If audit activity is well staffed and well managed then audit officers will take over most of the burdens of clinicians, who will be able to spend their time on design of audit, setting standards, and initiating changes highlighted as being necessary. This is why it is so important that audit officers are not side tracked (whether by clinicians or by management) into other activities such as writing computer programs, having to pull patients' notes, secretarial work, data input, or research. In this regard, it is worth deciding who pulls the notes before the appointment so that the new officer isn't faced with irate or intractable medical records staff, as we know has happened frequently.

In some regions a regional audit coordinator has been appointed, again with several roles. One of us (JF-C) has a background in research, clinical psychology, and organisational development, and her role is the facilitation of audit—getting it going—largely through workshops, evaluation of change, and coordinating medical audit with the introduction of audit by other professional groups. The other (PV) has a background in nursing and audit,

91

and her role is providing expertise to those undertaking regional audits and providing training for audit officers throughout the district. How these posts are defined will depend very much on local need and know how.

What do audit officers need?

Even in regions in which the appointment of audit officers was deferred until there was clearly a role for them, we still hear of first days in the job with nothing to do, no office, no clear relationship with anyone. There is often a temporariness about their posts which must be hard to take: accommodation in portacabins, no office cleaning, refusals to supply stationery, no recognition by the switchboard, or exclusion from the circulation list. This is largely because many officers are on short term contracts and all are funded with ringfenced money, which seems to give them an ephemeral quality. It certainly does seem to fulfil the intentions of the Department of Health that audit is here to stay and that its funding will eventually be provided for through contracts.

Most audit staff relate to the chairperson of the district audit committee (or its equivalent since 1 April 1991) for their work and to someone in management, information, or quality for their working conditions. The fewer the audit officers employed, the more support the chairperson should provide: the job can be lonely and, with its newness, it can be both vague and difficult. Again, we have heard of great variation in this relationship: from officers who rarely meet the chairperson, except at formal meetings, to a chairman who hangs his coat in the person's office and does most of his audit activity from there. Certainly chairpersons will find that they retain these valuable audit staff more easily if they put their weight behind getting such staff decent accommodation and ensuring that their duties are regarded as a part of the hospital's day to day activity.

Now that money has been given to regions separately for the inception of clinical audit—by nurses and other professional groups—it seems important that audit officers should be used more widely, when appropriate, rather than separate audit empires being established, which will be detrimental to audit itself and to the staff involved. Where local clinical audit committees are being established, consisting of medical and other professionals, it seems less likely that this will occur, and this generally must be a more fruitful progression.

Training needs

One question which should be addressed is that of who will determine the training needs of audit officers. Ideally, of course, the officers themselves should identify these needs to the chairperson or the district audit committee. This, however, requires establishing a culture in which asking for training is seen as a positive action rather than a deficiency.

Many courses are springing up around the country, providing national training on topics both broad and narrow, and feedback on their quality varies wildly. A different approach, which might in the long term prove more fruitful, is where regions have set up local initiatives which, after an introductory course, aim at allowing the participants to design their own future syllabus according to their particular development needs. From such a programme we have seen requests for less predictable audit topics such as assertiveness training, medical terminology, and budgeting skills for those who find themselves involved in handling financial aspects of the job.

Conclusion

Audit, whether medical or clinical, is here to stay; our experience, young as it is, already suggests that audit flourishes best when well motivated and well cared for audit staff are employed. The more fully they are allowed to participate in the audit activity the better motivated they will be, and the more integrated they are into the hospital or community setting the more likely it is that they will stay and make audit work.

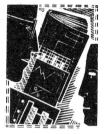

When medical audit starts to count

DAVID BOWDEN, KIERAN WALSHE

Medical audit has been the least controversial element of the NHS reforms. Its widespread acceptance by clinicians has been encouraging, though it is not surprising that organised medical audit is becoming part of everyday practice for the medical profession. Most clinicians have a genuine desire to prove to themselves and to others that they provide a high quality, effective service. That sense of altruism must never be allowed to diminish.

With a few notable exceptions,[1][2] however, previous medical audit activities in many hospitals were spasmodic, ad hoc, and uncoordinated. Recent extension and formalisation of audit in most specialties is encouraging because in future medical and clinical audit will be of vital importance to the fate of provider organisations. Whether they succeed or fail will depend not only on their quality of service but also on their ability to prove their effectiveness in terms of outcomes. That is when medical audit will really start to count.

But as medical audit becomes more central to the other major changes in the way the NHS is organised and managed, it in turn will need to be organised differently. There will be an inevitable move towards clinical audit involving other professionals within the clinical team. Medical audit will be more closely linked to risk management. There will be an imperative to relate quality of care with quantity and cost. More explicit quality standards and outcome measures will be specified in contracts between health authorities and their providers. Doctors and managers will be required to share medical audit information within agreed rules of confidentiality, and, generally, managers will want to show the value of their being involved in the audit process. The box outlines

Past and future characteristics of medical audit

Characteristic	Past	Future
Participation of doctors	Entirely voluntary, so dominated by enthusiasts	Almost compulsory, through peer pressure, job plans, clinical directorates, and contracting process
Participation of other healthcare professionals	Limited participation, except perhaps in data collection	Widespread participation in planning systems and collecting and analysing data
Participation of managers	Little management involvement or interest	Audit central to management objectives; managers involved and interested
Planning and development of audit systems	Uncoordinated, led by individual doctors, lacking comparability	Coordinated by clinicians and managers. Integrated with general information strategies
Resources for medical audit	Little explicitly allocated—dependent on individual commitment	Resources explicitly allocated—both direct and indirect costs recognised
Relevance to organisation's objectives	Peripheral to objectives as defined by review process, authority policies, etc	Central to organisation's objectives, as defined by contracting process. Important for organisation's viability/success
Effect on organisation's performance	Little effect on performance—few changes in individual or group clinical working practices	Measurable and continuing effect on organisation's performance—clinically and managerially

Modified from *Health Service Journal* 1989:1249 and reproduced with permission the changes in the characteristics of medical audit which are likely to take place.

Up to now managers have largely watched the development of medical audit from the sidelines, partly because of clinicians' sensitivity about the issue and partly because of managers' preoccupations with a wealth of other changes occurring in the past few years. But as medical audit becomes more important to how they manage their organisation, managers will not be content to be spectators; they will want to be players in a genuine partnership with clinical colleagues. They will need to identify what they can and should do to support the audit process and what they will expect and need from audit in the future.

What managers should do for audit

Environment

General managers have a responsibility to provide the right environment for audit, and, where it does not exist, an obligation to take the lead by giving top level commitment to developing a formal audit process. The experience in this health authority over seven years[3] suggests that an incremental, evolutionary and non-punitive, and participative peer review approach is more readily accepted than a system imposed by management. The clinician-manager alliance is therefore crucially important, as is a positive and proactive management style.

The health authority (in the case of directly managed units) or the NHS trust board also has an important role. Not only must it endorse and support the clinical audit initiative but it must also define its priorities in relation to the controversial quality versus quantity argument.[4] We believe that for those patients who are admitted to hospital the quality of care must not be compromised, even though the overall quantity of treatment and service consequently may be less. This issue surely must be addressed in all hospitals and other units, and a clear policy must be formulated.

Resources

Audit cannot be undertaken sensibly and comprehensively without proper support and allocated resources. The creation of new consultant job plans provides the ideal opportunity for managers to acknowledge the importance of audit by allocating specific sessional time for it as well as set times during the week for senior and junior clinicians to audit their work. This, in turn, will mean the quality-quantity trade off will be made more explicit, maybe with the consequence that previously worked clinics or theatre sessions are forfeited. Resources are also needed to pay for specific research activities and for study leave. Funds must be made available to purchase the necessary information systems and to provide technical and administrative support staff. Medical audit should not, therefore, be seen as a cheap, peripheral activity. It needs time, staff, and money to develop a proper, comprehensive approach. Of course such investments must be shown to result in improved outcomes and better patient care, as well as making the work of clinicians more professionally rewarding.

Information systems

Information systems are a key tool in audit. As the volume and complexity of medical audit activity increase, it will become important that the information needs of medical audit are integrated into corporate information strategies. While the sense of clinical ownership of the information must not be lost, medical audit activities, resource management, contracting, and other management processes will benefit from the use of a shared database.

Incentives for audit

The new contracting mechanism will provide incentives for providers to meet agreed workload targets at lower overall costs than the specified contract price without affecting adversely the quality standards identified. This may be achieved by developing more efficient systems of working, and when costs are reduced the funds saved should be able to be retained for use by the clinical departments concerned. Similarly, we should now be looking at ways to create systems of incentive to reward clinicians achieving proved improvements in clinical outcomes, with the emphasis on recognising improved performances rather than imposing sanctions to penalise under-achievers.

Techniques

Together, clinicians and managers should be developing and facilitating the introduction of new techniques in audit, such as

Rights of access of different staff groups to medical audit information

Staff	Information on care or treatment of one patient		Aggregate information on care and treatment of a group of patients	
	Consultant or clinical team identified	Consultant or clinical team not identified	Consultant or clinical team identified	Consultant or clinical team not identified
Consultant or clinical team involved	Complete	Complete	Complete	Complete
Consultant colleagues of consultant or clinical team involved	If agreed by consultant involved	Complete	If agreed by consultant involved	Complete
Consultant manager or clinical director for service in which consultant works	Complete	Complete	Complete	Complete
District Medical Audit Advisory Committee (DMAAC) or similar body	Not normally required	Not normally required	Complete	Complete
Unit or district general managers	Not allowed	Not allowed	As agreed by DMAAC	As agreed between DMAAC and management*

*Unit and district general managers will be given details of the District Medical Audit Advisory Committee's forward programme, an annual report of progress within the district, and regular reports which will be sufficiently detailed to assure them that effective audit is taking place and to identify areas where management action might improve the quality of care.

adverse occurrence screening,[5] random record review, and criterion based audit,[6] as well as focused audit studies and an agreed approach to external accreditation and review.

Peer review audit and patient satisfaction

Managers are required, where necessary, to provide the interface between standard setting based on internal peer review (looking at patient care from within the organisation) and standards of patient satisfaction (looking at the organisation from outside). They should be involved in helping to reconcile the potentially conflicting viewpoints of clinicians and patients on some issues.

Confidentiality

With litigation for medical malpractice increasing in frequency, general managers have a responsibility to establish guidelines on confidentiality of medical information within the organisation and outside it. The guidelines should have the twin aims of preserving clinical confidence and using audit information properly. The table shows a model developed by Brighton Health Authority and South East Thames Regional Health Authority for determining the rights of access of different staff groups to medical audit information.[7]

In summary, managers must give a lead, and provide appropriate staffing, funding, and support, to make it easier and more rewarding for clinicians to perform their duties. They should not seek to interfere with doctors' individual clinical judgments but rather to maximise the extent of clinical freedom enjoyed by medical and other professional staff. This is best achieved by managers and clinicians working more closely as partners.

What managers expect and need from medical audit

Access to information

Managers in both commissioning authorities and provider units need information to determine the quality of the clinical services provided and to assess which clinical activities and treatments actually produce the most effective outcomes. That information should not only identify the standards related to the processes used in the departments concerned but, increasingly, compare the predicted and actual outcomes of those activities. Information is also required to allow managers to assess how well the audit

99

programmes are working and whether they are meeting the object-ive of producing better patient care. While most managers will be committed to supporting audit they will be reluctant to see resources devoted to it if it does not produce measurable benefits for patients.

Audit in contracting between purchaser and provider

Without doubt, the health authorities, as commissioners of clinical services, will establish progressively more advanced qual-ity standards in the service contracts they agree with provider hospitals and community services. General practitioner fund-holders will also have similar aims in their contracting process. This will force the providers to demonstrate not only that they have formalised audit programmes in place but also that they meet the jointly agreed treatment standards. Providers that cannot match these expectations may well not be asked to provide the services in the future.

Audit and managing the organisation

The inevitable development of clinical directorates will gradu-ally see the natural withering away of the cogwheel divisional committees. This will provide an increasingly more powerful position for doctors within the hospital or unit. They will be empowered with more control and authority for managing the resources used within their directorates, and collectively the clin-ical directors and consultant managers, as members of the unit management team, will influence much more directly the running of the whole organisation. The clinical director is pivotal to the management of the service as he or she combines professional knowledge with managerial clout. But the directors need medical audit information to support their decisions and actions. Audit has been the missing third leg of the resource management tripod which relates activity or workload to costs and quality. The general manager will expect to see all three elements being managed together within directorates, with medical audit and management of resources converging to provide real evidence of total value for money. The key to this is that the clinical director should be accountable for ensuring that there is a totally integrated manage-ment of quality, quantity, and cost. Cost effectiveness and clinical effectiveness must be linked. Running a directorate more efficiently both releases and generates more resources, which can be used to maximise clinical freedom. In many ways organisational arrangements are as important as individual clinical practices in determining the quality of service provided.

Audit involving other professionals

Medical audit is part of a matrix of quality assurance systems that includes a range of clinical professionals and assesses a range of aspects of quality of care. Lines of demarcation and strict professional boundaries make no sense; patients cross them all the time. As confidence allows, medical audit should gradually become part of a multidisciplinary, clinical audit system. This should not detract in any way from the importance of medical audit based on peer review, but there is much to be said for moving towards an audit system centred on patients rather than professions.

Audit and risk management

With the removal of Crown immunity and with Crown indemnity ensuring that the new provider organisations are legally responsible for all their care, they must seek to eliminate, or at least minimise, the risks to patients (of injury) and to the organisation (of litigation). Audit has a preventive role in this context and risk management is a natural extension of audit. Risk management programmes are designed to identify and reduce actual or potential risks to patient safety so that patient care is improved and negligence claims are restricted. General managers will wish to ensure that such programmes are developed and that medical audit systems relate closely to them.

In conclusion, medical audit is going to matter in future—to managers and clinicians in provider organisations, to commissioning authorities, and to patients. It will be crucial to the success and viability of providers in the new NHS, therefore managers and clinicians have to work together in provider organisations to develop their medical audit programmes. Doctors should seize this opportunity to be much more involved in shaping provider services, as a key part of a multiprofessional team. Managers should rise to the challenge of becoming better educated and better informed about the work of their clinical colleagues. Between them they can make medical audit start to count.

1 Buck N, Devlin HB, Lunn JN. *Report of a confidential enquiry into perioperative deaths.* London: Nuffield Provincial Hospitals Trust and King's Fund, 1987.
2 Gruer R, Gunn AA, Gordon DS, Ruckley CV. Audit of surgical audit. *Lancet* 1986;i:23–6.
3 Gumpert R, Lyons C. Setting up a district audit programme. *BMJ* 1990;**301**:162–5.
4 Bowden D, Gumpert R. Quality versus quantity in medicine. *Journal of the Royal Society of Arts* 1988:333–46.
5 Bennett J, Walshe K. Occurrence screening as a method of audit. *BMJ* 1990;**300**:1248–51.
6 Shaw C. Criterion based audit. *BMJ* 1990;**300**:649–51.
7 Walshe K, Bennett J. *Guidelines on medical audit and confidentiality.* Bexhill on Sea: South East Thames Regional Health Authority, 1990.

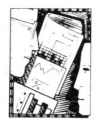

MAKING AUDIT HAPPEN

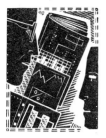

Defining essential data for audit in general practice

F DIFFORD

Medical audit may be defined simply as looking at what we are doing with the aim of making improvements in patient care and use of resources. Unlike research data, audit data are not intended to prove a hypothesis and require only as much scientific rigour as is needed to convince the participants of the kinds of changes needed. Audit is not a project in the sense that it has no end; the same audit may be repeated to check that the improvement is maintained. Data for audit should ideally therefore be continuously available as part of the process of care. Also, audit is not assessment that measures ability rather than performance, but the two are often confused because potential is commonly assessed by looking at what has been done. Recognition and promotion of this distinction is important in accepting the delegation of data handling. Audit is essentially looking backwards, and as none of the past can be changed audits should be small with only as many case studies as are required to produce valid findings. The data gathered for audit are transient and the details are of no value once conclusions have been drawn.

The nature of data for audit varies from objective numbers to subjective judgments depending on the topic examined. We may look at the basic structure of provision of care, at clinical processes, and at various outcomes for patients. Table I shows topics for audit, suggested examples, and the type of data required. In topics such as consultation and audit of deaths and new morbidity much will be quite subjective or debatable. Imagination is needed in meeting the challenge that the most important things are not measurable. The rest of this article is confined to considering numerical data.

TABLE I—Topics for audit in general practice and sources of data

	Examples	Source of data
Organisation of practice	Availability of appointments	Record of appointments available per week, per day, and just before surgery
	Delay in appointment time	May be available on computer appointment systems
	Response time in emergency calls	Recording time of receipt of message and arrival time
Consultation skills		Videotape or audiotape analysis
Examination skills		Patient questionnaires
Manual treatment skills		Outpatient clinics
Management of an acute diagnosis, symptom, or sign	Urinary tract infection	Review notes to ascertain diagnosis
	Vertigo	Adherence to clinical protocol
		Numbers of patients
Management of chronic illness	Diabetes	Glycated haemoglobin/fructosamine concentrations
		Recording of weight, etc
Screening	Hypertension	Numbers with blood pressure recorded in past three years
Immunisation	Immunisation rates in children	
Use of investigations	x Ray examinations	All x ray examinations in past three months
Outpatient referral		No of patients over six months in chosen specialties
Inpatient referral		
Domiciliary consultations		
Private referral		Total numbers
Referral to other than consultants		
Prescribing		Indications for prescribing given drug to individual patients
Premature death		Complete record of deaths
Avoidable morbidity		List of all new disabilities
Avoidable suffering		"Disaster board"

Defining and recording data

Much of the data for audit are best defined in protocols, which, ideally, should precede any intention to carry out audit but in practice are often the first stage. In a protocol we define what we think we should be doing—our objectives—and the processes to achieve them. The protocols may be organisational or clinical and may be based on personal decisions or agreed in the practice or on a more widespread basis. Although a broad measure of unwritten agreement exists on objectives, many written protocols seem to fail by attempting to gain a consensus that is too detailed clinically. The more widespread the protocol used, the more basic it and the ensuing audit need to be. Objectives are often expressed as criteria (for example, all patients aged over 75 should be interviewed about their repeat treatment every 12 months) and a level of performance (or "target"), set as the percentage of patients in whom this can be achieved. Criterion and performance together constitute a "standard," and the process of reaching agreement is referred to as standard setting. Doctors often seem to set unrealistic standards, taking little account of the time available or patients' compliance. More overall clinical benefit may ensue by reaching more patients at less frequent intervals, so that by changing the criterion more time is released to reach a wider population.

Auditing an entire area defined in a protocol is not necessary. The number of variables examined should be limited to, at most, half a dozen to give time to audit other areas and so help prevent subconscious rejection of difficult subjects. The problem here is that repeated audits of the same variables inevitably lead to a concentration on getting these right. Objective measurements such as "visual acuity 6/36" are more reliable than "fundi OK" in auditing management. Ideally, data should be recorded as part of the routine provision of care as any temporary recording methods are likely to induce only temporary changes in behaviour. Audits that result early in newly designed encounter sheets or follow up cards have often become projects to implement changes in a particular area and though commendable in themselves, they have displaced the auditing process. Data should ideally be gathered by ancillary staff so that the doctors' work is confined to analysing them and effecting necessary changes. Some data will uncover omissions on individual patients that might be corrected immediately. This incidental activity should not distract from the main purpose of audit, which is to determine whether special measures are required for improvements—in time, resources, or education. To decide this we can compare our results either with previous identical audits in the same practice or with audits in other practices, in which case the comparison is valid only if the data are defined identically, which is best achieved by using identical protocols. Variations among practices such as in age and sex distribution should be taken account of in the protocol, but when social deprivation exists or levels of community resources differ it may have to be accepted that no comparison is possible and separate protocols are required.

Population denominators

A complete population denominator is essential for providing accurate data for audit, whether this is the entire age and sex register or individual cohorts. Computers have now the potential to provide the most accurate register of the population. New contractual arrangements may provide a solution to the problem of "ghost" patients, for if a patient who has not been seen for three years cannot be contacted for a three year assessment then the general practitioner is obliged to notify the family practitioner committee and, presumably, the patient will be removed from the doctor's list. In any case this patient cannot be part of an audit denominator. Another problem arises with newly registered patients for whom it is impossible to meet an audit criterion if the previous general practitioner has just met the criterion, or if the notes are slow to arrive, or if the patient has been living in the practice area for several years without registering. A solution is to exclude such patients from the audit population for the audit period, although they would of course be part of the population to which the service is provided. Thus a general practitioner looking at his or her screening for blood pressure in the past three years should not include patients newly registered within that time. This may become increasingly necessary if patients change doctors more frequently with the change in regulations. With computers any figures based on sex and age may be converted into those that apply to the standard national population, but for most practices the difference is probably not large enough to matter. If we can define social class or occupation in the computer register it may be possible to audit the uptake of services among social classes.

Similarly, a complete cohort of patients is essential for audit of chronic diseases. Thus unless an audit is of diabetics who attend only the practice clinic or it specifically excludes diabetics attending outpatient clinics it should include all identified diabetics in the practice and not omit those who are seen infrequently. Manual disease registers or, preferably, disease indexes in computers can provide a more complete list and a statistical calculation may be made about the completeness of the list. If there are too few diabetics there may be a basic flaw in the audit. Obtaining a complete audit of acute illnesses is more difficult because there are less presentations to record and they may easily be omitted. The increasing use of computers in consultation allows presentations to be identified, provided that doctors use agreed codes for recording.

Data for audit may be a complete descriptive analysis or based on random sampling. Total descriptive audits are possible with computers, even when large numbers are concerned. Computer protocols have now been developed that search the electronic record for areas of preventive care or chronic disease management that are due for review and prompt the doctor about the missing data and provide an easy means of updating the computer record. The same protocols may be audited automatically by the computer. While most practices, however, still regard computers as only helping the manual record, the data held on them are commonly incomplete, and sampling of the manual record may be more reliable. Computers provide a ready method of random sampling and are able to carry out necessary statistical calculations as data are produced. Some argue that computers will remove the need for sampling, but there will always be aspects of audit that need a closer look than computer technology makes possible, and we will want to do this on a sample. How, for instance, do you decide that treatment has been reviewed?

The duration of data analysis required for valid results needs consideration in those studies which audit events, such as the use of x rays and referrals. Within the average practice quite large variations occur and make it misleading to look at a set of three months' figures. Referral figures are best considered by looking at individual specialties, but in some specialties the small numbers concerned may mean taking several years together before any conclusions may be drawn. In contrast, when numerous events may be involved, such as laboratory investigations, a random sample over a longer period may give a truer picture than every test over a few weeks. Once again, these figures are becoming readily available with computers. In particular it is possible to obtain a report on all prescribing of a particular drug or group of drugs over a chosen period and then refer to all the individual records for the reasons for prescribing.

External sources of data

Data for audit are also available from outside the practice. Thus family practitioner committees may analyse claim forms—for example, numbers of patients receiving contraceptive care, number of visits between 11 pm and 7 am, and numbers of ancillary staff employed. For the most part these types of data result in audit on the completion of claim forms rather than the provision of a service, but numbers of staff employed is a useful audit of structure in the practice. District health authorities have a well defined set of performance indicators that contrast sharply with the variety of data for audit in general practice suggested here and elsewhere. But these indicators are concerned mainly with large scale finance and administration and have little relevance to the individualism of doctor and patient in the community. We have something similar in the prescribing analysis and cost data and proposed "indicative" drug budgets, in which most of the analysis is in terms of costs. The term "indicator" implies that there is not a target and that underprescribing could be occurring as well as overprescribing. In due course the district health authorities will be able to produce the referral, admission, and investigation rates for individual general practitioners, which again will be indicators rather than targets. As already seen in prescribing analysis and cost data interpretation of these figures is reliable only at the practice level and may be unreliable for individual doctors because of recording errors and variations in workload and case mix. We do now have a defined target for cervical cytology (table II) as well as the long established target of 90% for childhood immunisation.

These indicators and targets comprise a contractual audit. Unfortunately general practitioners may be so occupied meeting their obligations under this audit that they will not appreciate the difference between it and audit led by the profession, the most important part of which is considering the results and learning how to improve, and this is best done in an educational setting.

TABLE II—Example of computer audit of cervical cytology in this general practice, 17 May 1984–16 November 1989

	Code	No*	%
Women:			
Aged 25–64 years now		2221	
With hysterectomy		195	9
Cervical smear result	.4K2	1580	77·99
Cervical smear result	4K2.	102	
Inadequate specimen	4K21	20	
Negative	4K22	1479	
Mild dyskaryosis	4K23	29	
Severe dyskaryosis	4K24	22	
Severe dyskaryosis ? invasive cancer	4K25	11	
? Gland neoplasia	4K26	1	
Atrophic change	4K27	1	
Borderline changes	4K29	8	
Not otherwise specified	4K2Z	1	

*Each patient may have an entry in more than one category.

Recording data should be part of routine care provision and gathering data for analysis delegated whenever possible, leaving interpretation to general practitioners. The dramatic increase in the use of computers for clinical recording makes this the most valuable tool for future audit.

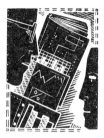

Defining essential hospital data

S J NIXON

The recent government white paper clearly states an intention that all doctors should be concerned with auditing the quality of patient care. No exceptions are made, and little advice is given to those who have no experience of audit. If audit is perceived as economy, efficiency, and effectiveness then the white paper emphasises the last of these three despite the view of some that the basis of government interest is that of cost cutting. The white paper's definition of audit avoids mention of cost savings but does indicate that improvements in the quality of care must be achieved within the "resources available." It clearly puts responsibility for audit within the medical profession, and this has been accepted by the royal colleges, which see a definite role for themselves as leaders in audit.

Audit is not new; the history of medicine contains many examples of people who have actively examined the quality of their practice. Collective audit, however, is a phenomenon of the twentieth century, and there are in the United Kingdom many outstanding examples of national audit of mortality such as maternal mortality, perinatal mortality, anaesthetic studies, and cardiac surgery. The confidential enquiry into perioperative deaths represents the most ambitious and in depth study yet undertaken. It may be insufficient, however, simply to join such studies in future. Doctors must look more closely into their own day to day activities.

Nature and quality of audit data

Audit has been subdivided into structure, process, and outcome. Structure has not been included in the remit of the white paper despite protests that it is clearly inadequate to meet the needs of patients. Though outcome is the most important, it is process that has been most subject to audit in the past because of simple, practical considerations. Data are most easily acquired while patients are in hospital or consulting rooms. Benefits of treatment are usually slow to accrue and need longer term assessment. Such follow up is time consuming, expensive, and often incomplete. The importance of outcome must, however, stimulate the profession to seek better methods for analysis of longer term results. Closer cooperation between hospital doctors and general practitioners might become the key to acquiring these data. Increasing use of computer technology in the community health service may be a catalyst to audit, but experience with hospital inpatient data suggests that useful audit as a byproduct of routine data capture is unrealistic.

Audit is research whose emphasis is on the quality of medical delivery rather than the basic principles of medical science. It is designed to influence "me" rather than "you." It must not be seen as second rate research. If poorly performed, audit will neither give a clear picture nor influence medical practice. Its data must be seen as a reliable indicator of the complex interaction between disease and treatment; too simplistic an approach will be dismissed by the profession. Data must also be collected and analysed rapidly for maximal effect.

Very real constraints on the quality and quantity of audit data exist. These include problems of definition, economics, time, and individual doctors' enthusiasm. Comparison of outcome depends on setting standards, which in turn relies on accurate predictors of diagnosis and severity of disease. Many studies show a high degree of variation in doctors' analyses of the same clinical data, resulting in differing views on severity of illness and diagnosis. There have, however, been many successful attempts to predict outcome—for example, the Glasgow coma scale, injury severity score, and prognostic formulas for predicting recurrence of various cancers— all of which have found international acceptance value. Little scientific study has examined prediction of outcome in more common situations—for example, repair of inguinal hernia, in which reported recurrence rates vary 100-fold from 0·2% to 20%. General surgeons need to look little further than surgery for hernia if they wish to define their position within this range. There are published methods designed to predict major complications and death after general surgical procedures. These still require wider verification but may help in setting standards of practice in future.

Coding systems

Audit requires the ability to compare results with those of colleagues, and this demands coding systems of disease, severity, and outcome. Sadly, the history of diagnostic and operation codes suggests that in surgery we still do not have a coding system that doctors use in day to day practice. Read codes may solve this problem. In Lothian surgeons devised their own coding of diseases and operations, which was developed specifically for audit and took five years to develop before being introduced in 1984. The coding is used by all general surgeons working in the area and has spread to other areas. It has been used to acquire data on over 200 000 operation procedures but requires annual modification to keep pace with changes in practice. In urology so great have been the recent changes that a complete revision has been undertaken. It does show, however, that coding systems can be made "doctor friendly" if working doctors are involved in their development.

As an indicator of outcome death remains the most studied and universally accepted; matters of definition do not arise. There are many areas of medical practice in which mortality is still relevant and in which wider variations seem to occur within the United Kingdom than can be explained by case mix alone. British reports of mortality for colonic resection vary from 0% to 33%. Interestingly, mortality in Lothian has fallen from 10% to 5% during the 1980s, when colonic surgery has been much discussed by the surgeons there, and it compares favourably with that in similar published work. The confidential enquiry into perioperative deaths confirmed large variations in the proportion of deaths considered to be "avoidable." A call by hospital adminstrators that hospital mortality be published may be premature as the analysis of such data is open to misinterpretation, but more detailed study of variations in mortality seems appropriate.

The lead taken by surgical audit is often dismissed as simply due to the relative ease of counting operations, complications, and deaths. I see little difficulty in analysing myocardial infarction, stroke, haematemesis, and many other conditions that are as clearly defined as an operation and with equally clear end points. I also see great problems in auditing some types of medical practice. Within surgery inflammatory bowel disease is representative of those conditions with a highly unpredictable course. With our present state of knowledge such conditions are simply not within the scope of audit and should be avoided.

As the momentum to audit increases there will be a temptation to overambition. Lothian surgical audit has been set as an example for others. It collects basic data from all operations and all deaths and has established a foundation of reliable data. Its data set is, however, limited and its methodology simple. It collects data from working documents and is seen as non-threatening and basically educational. It has evolved over 40 years to its present state and has proved to be a major stimulus for change in Lothian, usually towards increased specialisation; I doubt that any surgeon in Lothian has been immune to its influence. The Scottish mortality study is expanding this data set and attempting to establish the level of data collection that surgeons and anaesthetists will tolerate. The confidential enquiry into perioperative deaths is taking the alternative approach of collecting detailed data from a narrow field study. All of these studies illustrate that successful audit must have limited objectives if wide compliance is to be assured.

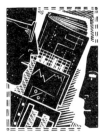

Random review of hospital patient records

D A HEATH

In 1978 the departments of medicine and clinical pharmacology of Birmingham University instituted a regular weekly medical audit meeting. Details of the meetings and the effects of audit have been previously described.[1][2] Basically, notes were chosen randomly from inpatient admissions once the final discharge summary had been completed. The notes of one consultant firm were then reviewed by another consultant firm, which commented on various points, including the quality of the notes at admission and follow up, appropriateness of investigations and drug treatment, speed of producing discharge summaries and their content, and evidence of communication among staff, patient, and general practitioner. These meetings were held regularly and successfully for many years. During the hour devoted to audit each week two sets of notes were analysed for each consultant firm and hence only a fraction of the total number of inpatients managed by the firm were reviewed. This style of audit has now been introduced throughout all medical firms in this hospital, primarily as a result of the decision of the Royal College of Physicians of London to make audit an essential feature of junior doctor training.

In this article I will discuss the advantages and disadvantages of this form of audit as practised by the original four consultant firms and now by 14 consultant firms. The views are mine and do not necessarily reflect those of my colleagues.

The advantages of the original audit were that, as practised, it was simple to do and entailed little administrative time, and no computers or additional staff were required as the secretaries merely choose at random two sets of notes for which a discharge summary had recently been completed. As only four consultant firms were concerned notes from each firm were analysed at each meeting so that all staff present were involved in the meeting. This also meant that an appreciable proportion of the work of each firm was audited, perhaps 10–20% of all admissions.

The disadvantages were that most notes were not audited, so that major mistakes could easily be missed; no attempt was made to audit outpatient practice; and by auditing after the patients had left hospital, it was too late to alter their management. The process did not entail other groups involved in patient management—for example, nursing staff, general practitioners, etc. In fact, nursing staff attended some of the early meetings, but it proved impossible to arrange for them to leave the ward regularly to attend.

Lessons and achievements

Despite these disadvantages several important lessons were learnt and achievements attained. First and foremost, it became clear that audit could be practised in a friendly, non-confrontational manner in a form that was enjoyed by all who participated. Major mistakes were, in fact, uncommon and, when identified, were usually incomprehensible even to those who had made them. For instance, a patient of mine was prescribed spironolactone at a time when the serum potassium concentration was $> 6 \, mmol/l$. How could this happen? It had to mean that prescribing at times took place without reference to investigations. The identification of the mistake allowed the ward practice to be reviewed. Although in this example the prescription was unequivocally wrong, most discussions usually centred around the appropriateness of certain investigations or treatments, when there is often no absolute answer. This disclosed that much of our medical practice was often based on habit rather than medical facts. Often no unified conclusion emerged—for instance, there is no one correct way of investigating an elderly patient with an iron deficiency anaemia or a patient with a swollen leg. Almost imperceptibly, however, after several discussions of similar cases, policies started to change and become more uniform.

Initially, reporting of the illness and subsequent progress was poor; information on what had been said to patients regarding illness and progress in the inpatient notes and correspondence was almost non-existent. All these deficiencies improved immediately audit was instituted. Although it was possible to measure and show the benefit of audit on reporting in the notes and discharge summaries,[2] it was more difficult to do so for investigations and treatment and impossible for patient morbidity and mortality. The failure to show an effect of audit on investigations was at first sight disappointing but, on reflection, expected. The average general medical admission is an emergency admission with a condition that does not require extensive investigation and often settles rapidly—for example, asthma or heart failure—or, if not, requires long term management rather than prolonged investigation—for example, a dense stroke. To show an effect of audit on investigations I suggest that the elective investigation of a specific problem would need to be chosen. There are, however, few specific conditions regularly investigated by most doctors, making local comparisons difficult. The failure of this form of audit to have any demonstrable effect on outcome, has been leapt upon by some as an indication of the lack of benefit of audit and used to resist its introduction. It would be amazing, however, if this form of audit could be shown to affect, say, mortality in general medicine; you have only to think of the size of trials required to show an effect of treatment on survival after a myocardial infarction. No one city, let alone one hospital or one consultant, could expect to show significant effects of management on morbidity or mortality after, say, a haematemesis, asthma attack, stroke, or overdose unless gross medical mismanagement was regularly taking place.

Once the meetings were well established and the problems of reporting dealt with, a problem of repetitiveness occasionally arose. One final point to emerge was that for audit to continue to be valuable it had to be supported by consultants who believed in its benefit and who were regular attenders.

Re-emergence of hospital audit

The directive of the royal college that medical audit must be seen to be taking place in hospitals training junior staff has led to the re-emergence of audit in this hospital, this time involving all physicians, both general and specialised. An identical format is being used, but the participation of all types of physicians has brought advantages and disadvantages. The disadvantages are the difficulty of finding a suitable time for all consultant teams to meet; also the increased participation of other firms automatically reduces the proportion of case notes examined in each firm to a low value. Currently, we meet each week and two firms are audited, meaning that any one firm will be audited every two months. The disadvantages have to be balanced by the participation of firms who previously did not conduct audit and by the ability to have specialist opinions on most topics.

Despite initial protestations the meetings have been well attended and some initial doubters have admitted to their value. Particularly encouraging has been the recognition by some of the consultants that now audit has to be done it is in our interest to try to do it properly. Most weeks it is considered that at least one important problem that warrants attention is unearthed. Of particular interest to me is the discovery of common practices that are unknown by most of the consultants despite the fact that they were occurring on their firms—a recent example being that most patients admitted to the hospital with a chest infection were having blood cultures performed. Now that the audit process has been accepted by the physicians it is clear that the format of future meetings will need to be changed. A mechanism needs to be set up to ensure that queries or problems identified at the meetings are properly researched or followed up. To this end it is planned to have nominated consultants to do this and to report back to subsequent meetings. Several of the laboratories and support services have asked to be present at meetings to discuss the way they are being used or misused by the clinicians. They can be incorporated into the rota, and this will help to maintain the interest of the meetings.

Although I have had it pointed out that the random case review seems to be directed almost exclusively at looking for mistakes and does not seem to want to record how well we practise medicine, it seems to me to be far more important to become aware of the occasions that we perform inefficiently or badly rather than applaud those when we do well, which we inevitably recognise anyway. Our current method is guaranteed to miss most problems. However, the principle of audit is to try to make doctors think constantly about why they are doing things and may in itself lead to a reduction in errors. Despite this it would be a major advantage to identify cases in which errors are more likely to have occurred. Concentrating only on deaths is unlikely to be worthwhile as most are unavoidable. Certain categories might be identified for automatic review—for example, all deaths under 40, deaths after gastrointestinal bleeding, those after asthma, etc. Another strategy is the process of severity adjusted analysis.

Selecting cases for audit

The length of time that a patient stays in hospital depends on various factors; primarily, it depends on the illness and is also influenced by any other coexistent diseases, so that a patient with chronic liver disease who has gastrointestinal bleeding is likely to need a longer stay in hospital than one without. Average times that any patient might be expected to stay in hospital may be calculated for a series of primary conditions, and these can be modified for the confounding effects of age and other classified disorders present. The practice of a hospital can then be examined and patients identified who stayed in hospital for a longer than expected period. Such patients will have stayed in hospital longer for various reasons, including complications of the disease (which may or may not have been preventable), personal policy of the management team, unavailability or poor use of facilities to permit efficient investigation of a problem, etc. These patients, if they can be selected, comprise a group that merits examination by audit and that is more likely to disclose problems that require identification than the random selection of patients who probably have had a short, uneventful stay in hospital. The surveillance of proper reporting can continue just as well on this selected group of patients.

Severity adjusted analysis is totally dependent on the proper and complete identification of the medical conditions present. This information at present should be collected to provide Körner data. Very little effort is made to check such data, and all the evidence is that it is often inaccurate or incomplete. Yet this information is currently being used to calculate the allocation of funds to different hospitals. If the data can be improved then evaluating severity adjusted analysis to see whether it really selects a group of patients who are more relevant for auditing should be possible. I hope that such a scheme at this hospital may be evaluated in the near future. This discussion of cases that have not progressed satisfactorily by specialists from many medical disciplines should permit the emergence of better practices. Such discussions would have a major educational role for both junior and senior doctors.

The decision of the college to expect audit to take place in all hospitals has given a massive impetus to developing proper auditing. I hope that its widespread introduction will have convinced non-believers that its primary use is to try to ensure a high level of patient care. It is not a weapon to save money or to punish doctors, and, used sensibly, it may help our medical practice rather than hinder it. Techniques of auditing are still in their infancy, and with wider experience different and better methods will be found; rather than resist or mock the present system it behoves the medical profession to support the development of audit and to improve patient care.

1 Heath DA, Hoffenberg R, Bishop JM, Kendall MJ, Wade OL. Medical audit. *J R Coll Physicians Lond* 1980;**14**:200–1.
2 Heath DA. Medical audit in general medicine. *J R Coll Physicians Lond* 1981;**15**:197–9.

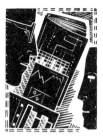

Criterion based audit

CHARLES D SHAW

Observations in Britain and overseas suggest that the introduction of medical audit seems to have fallen into four phases. In the first (philosophical) phase the debate is whether doctors should be involved, in the second (organisational) phase who should lead and what resources are required, and in the third (practical) phase what should be audited and exactly how; in the fourth (invasive) phase ideas on audit are disseminated through publications and education. This account focuses on the practical phase and the search for a simple method of audit that is applicable generally to medical and surgical specialties. It may therefore be useful first to define the principal characteristics that differentiate formal medical audit from traditional methods of clinical review (box).

Differences between audit and traditional review

● Use of explicit criteria for measurement rather than implicit judgments
● Numerical comparison of current practice patterns against these criteria
● Comparison of practice among peers
● Formal identification of action required to resolve any discrepancies disclosed
● Recording the process to retain information and increase impact of audit on future management.

Although some innovative methods have been described, which might be applied in hospital practice (such as reciprocal visiting[1] and videotape recordings of sample consultations[2]), audit techniques generally fall into one of three categories.

(1) Review of routine statistics and selected adverse patient events, including that of all predefined adverse events such as morbidity and mortality and of routinely collected statistics. This excludes most patients, who benefit from medical care without complications.

(2) Review of randomly selected records. Analysis of individual patient records by a senior doctor, with an agreed format gives valuable insight into objectively selected cases. Judgments of the "adequacy" of medical care, however, remain largely subjective.

(3) Review of a topic. Analysis of an agreed topic may be carried out by prospective study (which might include a survey of patient satisfaction) or by a retrospective analysis of medical records (which assumes that good practice is reflected by good records and that audit on this basis may approximate the two). Criterion based audit, widely adopted in North America, Australia, and The Netherlands, offers a realistic method of audit based on analysis of medical records despite their current elusive and inadequate state in the United Kingdom and less advanced computer systems.

Practical steps to criterion based audit

Step 1: choose a topic

The audit group should select a topic that is of general interest. To gain most benefit for time spent it is important to pick a topic that is significant either as being common, high risk, or high cost or as an issue of contention or local interest. It may be a diagnosis (such as schizophrenia or pulmonary embolism), an investigation (such as an intravenous pyelogram for haematuria), a treatment (such as palliative radiotherapy for carcinoma of the bronchus), or a general problem (such as chest pain in the accident unit). Locally relevant topics may arise from review of the routine statistics and by meetings on morbidity and mortality.

Step 2: choose criteria for screening records

The purpose at this stage is not to define a universal protocol for clinical management but to identify key elements in management, which should be apparent to a non-medical analyst from the medical records. These criteria are to allow large numbers of records to be screened so that only those records that fail substantially to meet them are selected for further clinical review. A limited number (12–15) of simple questions that can be answered either yes or no and that are self evident from the medical records should be defined. For an audit of inpatient care, for example, these questions may fall under the headings of:

Referral—The acceptable method or delay between referral and first contact with the specialist—for example, not more than four weeks between diagnosing carcinoma of the bronchus and starting palliative radiotherapy.

History—Reference to items essential in establishing a diagnosis—for example, the duration and radiation of chest pain in suspected myocardial infarction.

Examination—Essential clinical observations—for example, the type and distribution of rash in psoriasis.

Investigation—Reference to critical diagnostic tests—for example, lung scanning in pulmonary embolism.

Treatment—Evidence of agreed essential management—for example, administration of streptokinase within six hours after onset of chest pain in acute myocardial infarction.

Follow up—Critical decisions in the monitoring and modification of treatment—for example, the frequency of haematological monitoring and responsibility (consultant, junior doctor, or general practitioner) for deciding to discontinue anticoagulation after pulmonary embolism.

Outcome—Evidence that the initial objectives of intervention have been met—for example, return of an otherwise healthy subject to full function within an agreed time after elective surgery.

Communication—Evidence that relevant information is given promptly to patients, relatives, general practitioners, or referring consultants—for example, sending a discharge letter to the general practitioner within seven days after discharge, defining the diagnosis, what the patient was told, current treatment, and the arrangements for follow up.

The criteria should occupy no more than one page but may require a glossary to clarify certain points. These may include "allowable exceptions" and target levels of compliance. Before embarking on a full audit testing the criteria on six records or so may be valuable to ensure that the audit assistant has a chance of obtaining the required information. The group should agree on how many records should be selected and how recent they should be. For example, 20 consecutive admissions with the agreed diagnosis may be selected from those of the previous year for each firm.

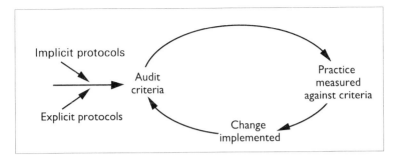

Linking audit with clinical guidelines

The process of choosing a topic and selecting criteria should take about one and a half hours, but the chairperson may need to attend to the wording of the criteria before giving them to the audit assistant who should, ideally, have been present at the meeting. Defining explicit criteria from the implicit judgment of each individual is an educational and challenging part of audit. It forces discussion and resolution of divergent opinions, which in many clinical meetings would remain unresolved. Often junior medical staff pose the most searching questions about how decisions are made and most appreciate an agreed common policy on patient management. It should be emphasised that this stage is merely for defining criteria for screening records; it is not for defining general policies of patient care. As the audit progresses, however, defining an explicit agreed protocol to replace several individual and implicit approaches to clinical management may become easier. The practical result of such an audit will therefore be a reconciliation of the existing protocols (either implicit or explicit) with what is shown to be actual practice (figure).

Step 3: analyse sample records

Analysing sample records is the most time consuming phase of criterion based audit but can be done by non-medical staff with the criteria developed as above and if non-medical staff are available to apply them. The total time required depends on how easily the records are recovered, the complexity of the criteria, and how many records are chosen for the sample. For example, 20 records from each of four firms may require 15 minutes each for analysis, which with time for retrieving and tabulating results might add up to 26 hours' technical time. This phase falls into four activities.

Identifying case numbers—Some form of case register is required to identify the record numbers of suitable patients according to procedure, diagnosis, or problems. All NHS hospitals can in theory produce such an index, but deficiencies in accuracy, completeness, and timeliness often lead clinicians to resort to ward books, theatre registers, and other manual systems—especially for outpatients.

Retrieval of case records—Of 94 records recently identified by a teaching hospital for audit, only 30 could be found, many of which were temporary folders for the most recent admission because the principal record could not be found. The extent of the problem varies among hospitals and departments, but the time required to retrieve records should not be underestimated. Indeed, the elusiveness of medical records may well be a valuable subject for audit.

Abstracting data—Each record is abstracted according to the criteria previously agreed, thus generating one completed sheet per case record.

Analysis of findings—The results of each firm are summarised on to a single sheet, which may include the numbers of records that differ substantially from the agreed criteria. An overall summary table presents the aggregate results of the four firms but does not include any identification of individual patients. The aggregate results are circulated to each firm before the second audit meeting.

Step 4: discussion of results

The discussion of results tends to include questions on the validity of the criteria chosen and on the significance of compliance or non-compliance. For example, should the criteria be adjusted to fit current practice or vice versa? Specific issues of administrative and clinical management that arise from the differences in patterns of practice—usually greater than expected—should lead to explicit decisions on policy changes; these should make clear who would be responsible for following through the recommendations. The conclusions do not often relate to shortage of resources (but if so would provide a cogent argument for funding); more often they concern the organisation of work (for example, the value of traditional hospital discharge summaries) or clinical decision making (for example, the use of chest radiography in suspected pulmonary embolism).

The chairperson should maintain a record of the participants, the general subjects discussed, the conclusions reached, and the action to be taken (no more than one A4 page), not only as a record for the specialty but also as a means of advising the district audit committee and any other medical colleagues. It would also constitute an adequate record for demonstrating audit to obtain recognition for training posts and to assure managers of effective internal review. The working papers that identify individual cases should be destroyed.

Step 5: repeat audit

It is important to agree in advance when the audit should be repeated to identify whether the agreed changes have been made and whether the original audit made any impact on clinical practice and management. As the criteria have already been agreed repeating the audit is fairly simple but requires technical time.

Discussion

This approach to audit may seem cumbersome, but it permits an objective and systematic approach without undue demands on clinician time, assuming that technical assistance is available. Criterion based audit is applicable to almost any clinical circumstance and can readily include practical issues of communications among doctors, clinical organisation, clinical decision making, efficiency of care, and the satisfaction of patients with their management and the information available to them. The use of explicit criteria "reduces to a minimum the use of healthcare professionals whose time is exceedingly costly, and whose interest in the review process is less than enthusiastic."[3] Jessee pointed out the added advantages of objectivity, the ability to examine process and outcome of care simultaneously, and the greater potential for influencing change, compared with normative comparisons.[4] If this method were rotated with others in a regular programme including meetings every fortnight any specialty would be unlikely to cover more than three criterion based audits within a year, including time for follow up. This would require an audit assistant for between 150–200 hours/year, even assuming that he or she were not busy with any other related activities.

In conclusion, criterion based audit fulfils the requirements of many doctors, particularly in non-surgical specialties, for a method that is objective, yields quantitative data, and is repeatable. It is important that doctors identify the resources they require for audit and how they propose to use them in a practical programme. The cost of recruiting and training audit assistants will certainly be less than the cost in opportunity of diverting clinicians from clinical practice. There is also therefore an economic argument for selecting criterion based audit rather than more traditional methods.

1 Royal College of General Practitioners. *What sort of doctor?* London: RCGP, 1985.
2 Coles C. Self assessment and medical audit: an educational approach. *Br Med J* 1989;**299**:807–8.
3 Donabedian A. Advantages and limitations of explicit criteria for assessing the quality of health care. *Milbank Memorial Fund Quarterly* 1981;**59**:99–105.
4 Jessee WF. Criterion based screening. *Identifying health care quality problems: a practical manual for PSROs and hospitals.* Chapel Hill: University of North Carolina School of Public Health, 1982.

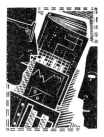

Retrospective review of hospital patient records

J G WILLIAMS, M J KINGHAM, J M MORGAN, A B DAVIES

Since March 1989 the medical division in West Glamorgan has held monthly district wide audit meetings, which are attended by the staff of all medical specialties from three district general hospitals. The chairman changes with each meeting, and the office rotates through all the consultants who attend. The chairman is responsible for researching and presenting an audit exercise of his or her choice. This system has resulted in much useful discussion of a broad range of topics.

Several criterion based studies, entailing retrospective reviews of hospital patient records, have been performed. These projects have provided insight into the difficulties associated with retrospective audit of case notes, and the lessons we have learnt are outlined below, with examples taken from an audit of the management of acute stroke.

Definition of objectives, criteria, and standards

A fundamental priority is to obtain agreement on the objectives of the project. A clear boundary and framework within which to work will help to keep the exercise manageable. The emphasis at this stage is on what to achieve, not on how to do it. Time spent on clear identification of the criteria to be assessed will be well used as mistakes are often made early and are difficult to correct later. Definition of standards may be difficult at this stage, and agreement may need to await discussion of the findings.

Objective—To audit retrospectively the current management of acute stroke in West Glamorgan.

Boundaries—All patients admitted to an acute medical or geriatric bed with a primary diagnosis of acute stroke from 1 October 1988 to a total sample of 200 patients.

Criteria—Delay to admission, selected findings on admission, use of computed tomography, recording of management decisions after investigation, treatment with aspirin, information given to patients' relatives before discharge, length of stay, and mortality.

Standards—Not defined at this stage.

Sample size

A brief feasibility exercise will show the time required to analyse each set of notes and will indicate the overall sample size that can be examined in the time available. If the population to be studied is large a limited sample (for example, by age or time) or random sample (for example, every 10th case note) may need to be selected.

Retrieval of case notes

A list of the identifying details of all patients falling within the boundaries of the study is compiled from administrative records or requested from an appropriate authority. Written permission will probably be required from all the consultants concerned.

The name, hospital number, date of birth, admission and discharge dates, and name of consultant in charge of patients admitted with a diagnosis of acute stroke were requested from Hospital Activity Analysis records held at the Welsh Office. Codes 436 and 342 of the International Classification of Diseases (ninth revision) were used.

A computer printout was received, with patients listed alphabetically and grouped by consultant. This created difficulties when requesting the case notes from medical records departments. Notes are filed numerically, in terminal digit order, and more efficient retrieval of the notes would have been achieved if the list had also been presented in this sequence.

Failure to retrieve some notes will be inevitable. This may cause a reduction in the total sample to be surveyed and will introduce bias if poor retrieval reflects different organisation, procedures, or efficiency among clinical firms. The notes of patients looked after by less efficient firms may be coded and returned to medical records less quickly and may therefore be underrepresented in the sample.

A few firms looked after most of the patients but yielded a minority of the notes retrieved because some patients were transferred to long term rehabilitation and a coded discharge summary was not produced until final discharge.

If a search is to be made according to diagnosis it is important to be clear whether this will be according to primary diagnosis alone or will include secondary diagnoses. Some notes may be wrongly coded on discharge. Elimination of such records may make the final target more difficult to achieve.

Of the notes retrieved, a fifth were inappropriate for the study: the diagnosis was from a previous admission (50% of these), a stroke had occurred after admission (30%), or in the wrong time period (18%), or the notes were wrongly coded (2%). A search according to primary diagnosis alone should have been stipulated. These factors and constraints of time necessitated a reduction of the sample size to 100 records.

Extraction of data

The order in which data are to be extracted from the notes should be logical and reflect the order in which information is recorded in clinical practice. Care must be taken not to make subjective judgments when information is assessed. This is best avoided by careful, agreed definition of the data to be extracted and strict categorisation of answers (for example, yes, no, insufficient information, or not recorded).

131

> The overall clinical state of the patient was poorly recorded in many cases, both on admission and on discharge, and there was a tendency for the reviewers to try to infer the clinical state from other information in the notes. In such circumstances clinical state should be recorded as "insufficient information" or "not recorded."

Time

A study of this type is labour intensive and takes time. Delays must be expected while awaiting authorising signatures from consultants and the list of patients. The time taken to find notes will vary among hospitals.

> It took nine days to collect signatures from the 14 consultants concerned and a further 32 days for the computer printout to arrive. Time taken to retrieve notes from medical records departments in the three participating hospitals varied from two to 16 days.

Bias

Incorrect coding on discharge, failure to retrieve notes, and differing rates of retrieval all contribute to bias the sample. If the patient list is in order of consultant and a fixed number of notes is to be assessed the differing rates of retrieval may be very important. Similarly, if notes are selected at random to limit numbers a high proportion of patients identified from smaller groups (for example, specialised clinic lists) will skew the sample.

> One of the criteria to be studied was length of stay, comparing care under general physicians and geriatricians. The Welsh Office printout showed that 30% were admitted under physicians and 70% under geriatricians. These proportions were reversed in the notes actually retrieved, invalidating any such comparison.

Analysis of data

Use of a computer with database, spreadsheet, and statistical or graphics software, or both, may greatly reduce time spent collecting, analysing, and presenting data, though smaller studies can be done without such help. If the questions to be answered have been carefully planned at an early stage final analysis and statistical testing should be straightforward.

> Standards were not predefined in this study. It was found that 30% of patients had had computed tomography, in some cases without clear indications. In itself this was not a useful statistic, but it was subsequently agreed that all patients meeting modified King's Fund criteria should be so examined.

Predefinition of criteria and standards will allow rapid filtering of those cases that do not require further examination. If standards have not been defined the exercise is more an evaluation of current practice, which, hopefully, will lead to consensus agreement on standards.

Checking for errors

There may be errors of subjective judgment, clerical transcription, or entry of data. If a computer system is used and the software is tailored for the project the degree of sophistication built into the human/computer interface is unlikely to be high as it would be difficult to justify the development time required to support a limited one off project. Consequently, it is vital to validate data and check for errors in extracting data, coding, and keyboard entry on a random sample.

> Ten sets of notes (a tenth of the total) were cross checked for errors. Considerable variation was found in the assessment of clinical state on admission and discharge due to subjective interpretation of inadequate clinical information. Coding and keyboard errors were not found.

Presentation and feedback

When the study is complete the results are presented for peer review. Simple overhead projector films or photographic slides are essential to summarise the data and provide prompts for discussion. The study protocol must be described clearly and the limitations of the method and areas of bias pointed out. A general overview of the results will need to be repeated with detailed discussion of each stage. Junior staff should be actively encouraged to participate in this discussion, which may require specific questions. Agreement of essential details will be easier if an independent chairman can mediate between the presenter and the discussants. Up to date, comprehensive knowledge of published work will permit an authoritative view of the subjects under discussion; without this there will be too much room for unsubstantiated comments that could prevent achievement of a consensus view. The meeting will need to be run at this stage with enough discipline to cover each item and then move on with at least majority agreement. The end result should be broad agreement on all the essentials of management, not forgetting those aspects that have not been discussed because they were not controversial. Ideally, the discussion should be minuted.

Written comments should be invited at the end of the meeting. The more shy, reserved, or polite members of staff may not speak. These written comments should be taken into account in producing a definitive protocol, which should be discussed with other affected parties (for example, radiologists) before its presentation, agreement, and distribution at the beginning of the next audit meeting.

The results of this exercise were presented at a district audit meeting attended by 45 people from across the medical disciplines. There was controversy over several aspects of management (for example, use of computed tomography, treatment with aspirin), which could not be resolved during the meeting without reviewing published reports. Subsequent feedback on paper added to the discussion, and final guidelines were issued at the next meeting. These will form the basis for criteria and standards for a future audit of acute stroke.

Conclusions

Retrospective review of hospital patient records can be a valuable audit exercise. It is time consuming, but careful preparation and analysis of requirements will ensure that this time is used effectively. It is important to acknowledge that the population of available records may not be representative of the true population, and recognition of causes of potential bias and allowance for them is more important than achieving a large, seriously skewed sample. A good retrospective study can also be a useful and cost effective feasibility exercise before setting up a long term prospective audit.

135

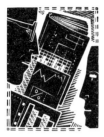

Problem solving with audit in general practice

RICHARD BAKER

Introduction

The purpose of medical audit is to improve the quality of care. If badly executed or used for any other purpose audit may waste time and resources that should be used in caring for patients. Whatever we may think of the other proposals in the white paper[1] the new arrangements for audit in general practice offer the profession an opportunity to introduce effective audit that will substantially improve the quality of care. The difficulty is to ensure that audit in practices or organised by medical audit advisory groups is effective in improving care and not wasteful of resources or demoralising to the participants. Audit should therefore be subjected to the same degree of critical evaluation as any other innovations in medicine, such as new treatments or forms of investigation; it has the same potential as these more traditional medical activities to cause harm as well as benefit. I will draw on the experience of some of the successful and unsuccessful audits carried out in my own practice to show why some audits lead to improvements in care and others do not.

Problem solving with audit

The most common reason for failure of audit to improve the quality of care is that the findings do not cause changes in day to day clinical practice. Deficiencies are ignored, either because they are seen as unimportant or because the changes required seem so considerable as to be impracticable. Using audit to solve problems is one way to avoid this difficulty; it is undertaken only when a problem is suspected, which the practice wishes to correct. If audit is to be effective the participants should be the practice team or some of its members—it is the practice that has the problem, and its members are usually the only people who can put it right.

Problems in providing care may be identified in various ways. There cannot be many general practitioners who are not aware of most of the strengths and weaknesses of the practices in which they work. For example, patients may complain about how difficult it is to speak to their doctor on the telephone or to arrange for repeat prescriptions. The receptionists or practice nurses may more often be the recipients of this type of complaint than the doctors themselves. There are other ways to spot problems. A potentially avoidable important event such as the late diagnosis of appendicitis may indicate a problem of practice management or medical skill that needs investigating; the information from prescribing analysis and cost data may show excessive prescribing of antibiotics; or a training practice inspection may disclose disorganised records. If the practice examines the evidence from such sources and concludes that a problem exists then audit provides one solution. Some types of audit can disclose deficiencies in care, but categorising those deficiencies as problems and then dealing with them demands a different approach. Deficiencies are not always acknowledged as problems. Problems can be thought of as deficiencies that those in the practice think are so important that corrective action must be taken. Some examples may help explain the difference.

Successful audits

Audit 1—The problem: doctors and staff reported to the practice meeting that patients complained how long they had to wait for routine appointments (urgent appointments are available on the same day). At the first data collection the receptionists kept a record of the waiting interval in days regularly over three months. The average wait for an appointment with the patient's chosen doctor was 3·7 days. The solution: we agreed to aim at around three days as a target and introduced a new system offering more and longer appointments. At the second data collection the average waiting time after introduction of the new system fell to 2·7 days during the three months of collecting data. Regular monitoring of waiting time continued subsequently; the percentage improvement in the problem was 27%.

Lessons: longstanding problems can be solved by a methodical approach; staff collected the data and the use of doctors' time was minimal.

Audit 2—The problem: during 1982 a large proportion of cervical smears were reported to the practice as inadequate, showing no endocervical cells. At the first data collection the practice nurse kept a record of the results. The proportion of adequate smears varied among the doctors from half (myself) to 78%. The solution: try harder, change fixative regularly, and buy better spatulas. At the second data collection, by 1983, my score had improved to 74% and is presently 87%, above the practice average of 83%. Percentage improvement in the first year was for myself 56% and overall 74%.

Lessons: audit may be embarrassing, but embarrassment is preferable to ignorance or lack of interest; audit works.

Audit 3—The problem: the district nurses asked during a team meeting whether giving hydroxycobalamin injections every month to patients with vitamin B-12 deficiency was an appropriate use of their time. At the first data collection a list of patients receiving hydroxycobalamin treatment was compiled from repeat prescriptions, the disease index, and the recall of team members. Records were reviewed, and all 32 patients receiving monthly injections were asked to change to three monthly injections. The second data collection was superfluous as the problem, according to the nurses, had been resolved. In terms of improvement 25 (78%) patients changed to the less frequent regimen.

Lessons: audit may help other members of the practice team not just the doctors. If the method that first disclosed the problem subsequently shows that the problem has been resolved repeating the audit cycle may be unnecessary.

Audit 4—The problem: achieving targets for preventive health measures for specific patient groups may be viewed as a problem, and many doctors have carried out problem solving audits of this type. Over several years our practice has tried to reduce the incidence of cardiovascular disease in our patients, one measure being a five yearly check on blood pressure for all adults aged under 65. At the first data collection in 1980, 52% of patients aged between 41 and 69 had their blood pressure recorded in their notes. We decided to rely on opportunistic screening. At the second data collection by 1983 the proportion had fallen to 38%. We reminded ourselves to check patients during consultations.

The first two sets of data were collected with a practice activity analysis method,[2] but thereafter we used our own method with larger samples of records. At the third data collection, in 1985, 60% of notes for the age group 35 to 65 had a record of blood pressure in the previous five years. A blood pressure check was routinely incorporated into the well woman screening scheme. At the fourth data collection by 1986 the proportion whose blood pressure was checked in the 35 to 65 age group was 60% for men and 65% for women. We decided to offer men health checks as well as continuing opportunistic screening and well woman checks. At the fifth data collection by 1989, 83% of men and 82% of women in the 35 to 65 age range had had their blood pressure recorded within the preceding five years.

Lesson: achieving a screening target may be treated as a problem to be tackled in a systematic way using audit combined with a concerted approach from the practice team.

Less successful audits

Audit 5—A study of referral to physiotherapy was carried out by an audit group of which I was a member. The group wanted to ascertain whether referrals were appropriate. At the first data collection over a two month period all members of the group kept a record of physiotherapy referrals. The doctor with the lowest number of referrals sent only one patient for treatment, the highest number of referrals was 11. No further data were collected. Percentage improvement was none.

Lessons: the senior physiotherapist told us that none of the referrals had been inappropriate. If we had asked her beforehand what proportion of referrals were inappropriate we would have realised that there was not a problem to audit.

Audit 6—The problem: participation in a trainer's course required me to perform a practice activity analysis study on workload. At the first data collection I learnt that I was doing more home visits but fewer surgery consultations than other participants on the course. No further data were collected and percentage improvement was none.

Lessons: this is an example of peer review. It might be thought of as educational, showing deviations from the average, but deviations are not always problems and no changes in my practice were brought about.

Audit 7—The problem: there was no specific problem but a general interest to perform a traditional audit of the care of patients with hypertension. At the first data collection in 1986 the records of a sample of patients with hypertension were reviewed; in 83% this hypertension was classified as being well controlled, while 4% had not been reviewed in the previous 12 months. We were reasonably happy with the findings but had not set any criteria or standards beforehand. At the second data collection in 1989 records were reviewed again; in 8% of patients in this sample hypertension had not been checked in the previous 12 months. We agreed to set a criterion that all patients should be seen at least annually. Percentage improvement was none.

Lessons: again this audit started out of curiosity rather than because of a specific problem. By finally agreeing a criterion, however, we defined a problem and set a target to encourage its resolution.

Differences between successful and unsuccessful audits

Successful audit leads to improvements in the quality of care. The audits described above show different degrees of success, those that resulted in improved care being initiated to deal with acknowledged problems. When set up for other reasons, such as compulsion or curiosity, they did not improve care. Peer review and audit for purely educational purposes are ineffective because they almost always tackle subjects most participants do not accept as problems, and even if they do their practices may not. Any deficiencies that are disclosed will not be corrected unless the practice agrees that they represent an important problem that must be corrected. There is a difference between deficiencies and problems. Deficiencies disclosed by chance or formal evaluations of care are deviations from standards that may or may not have been agreed beforehand. Problems are deficiencies that have been categorised by the members of the practice as needing action. The way in which a practice handles deficiencies and recognises them as problems will depend on the style of practice management, which needs an ordered way of considering problems and allotting a priority to each. In the multidisciplinary practice teams of today practice management must allow all professional groups to participate in identifying and resolving problems. If medical audit advisory groups are to encourage effective audit in general practice audit must be based in practices and used to solve deficiencies in care that each practice agrees are problems.

Some final advice

(1) As all good research starts with a clear hypothesis so good audit starts with a clear statement of the problem.

(2) If the results of the audit cycle cannot be expressed as a percentage improvement in the problem the audit was probably badly executed. (The most obvious exception is assessment of consultations.)

(3) Practice management and the team must be allowed to decide what is and what is not a problem.

(4) Whenever possible practice staff rather than doctors should collect data.

(5) Keep projects on a small scale and easy to repeat. Use samples. (Advice on sampling can be found in *Epidemiology in General Practice.*[3])

1 Secretaries of State for Health, Wales, Northern Ireland, and Scotland. *Working for patients.* London: HMSO, 1989. (Cmnd 555.)

2 Crombie DL, Fleming DM. *Practice activity analysis.* London: Royal College of General Practitioners, 1988. (Occasional paper 41.)

3 Morrell D, ed. *Epidemiology in general practice.* Oxford: Oxford University Press, 1988.

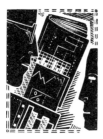

Occurrence screening as a method of audit

J BENNETT, K WALSHE

Brighton Health Authority has been actively pursuing a district wide quality assurance programme for almost five years since it first adopted a formal quality assurance strategy in 1985.[1][2] As part of that programme clinicians within the district, in cooperation with CASPE (Clinical Accountability, Service Planning and Evaluation) Research, have experimented with various approaches to medical audit. One of these techniques, developed in the United States and known as occurrence screening or screening criteria, has shown considerable promise and will form the basis of a hospital wide trial of medical audit at the district's main acute hospital.

Occurrence screening is based on two main principles: firstly, that it is far more practical to specify and describe what does not constitute good quality care than to specify what does; and, secondly, that focusing attention and resources on the investigation and analysis of instances of poor quality of care is an effective way to bring about improvement in overall standards of care. The specification and description of what does not constitute good quality care is set out in a set of screening criteria. The criteria are designed to highlight cases in which the patient experiences an adverse event or circumstance which, under optimal conditions, is not a natural consequence of his or her disease or treatment.[3] Such an event is sometimes termed an adverse patient occurrence.[4] Screening criteria may be generic or specific to particular specialties, conditions, or procedures. They are generally selected by the clinicians concerned with their use and may be based on clinical experience, empirical evidence, or academic research into what constitutes an adverse patient occurrence.

142

Date variation identified	Element	Date variation identified	Element
	1 Admission for adverse results of outpatient management		12 Other patient complications
	2 Readmission for complications or incomplete management on previous hospitalisation		13 Hospital-incurred patient incident: (a) Falls and accidents (d) Skin problems (b) IV problems (e) Equipment problems (c) Medication problems (f) Other
	3 Operative consent: (a) Incomplete (d) Different surgeon (b) Missing (e) Not signed by patient (c) Different from (f) No consent note procedure done (g) Other		14 Abnormal laboratory, radiographic, or other test results not accessed by physician
			15 Neurological deficit not present on admission
	4 Unplanned removal, injury, or repair of organ or structure during surgery, invasive procedure, or vaginal delivery		16 Transfer to another acute care facility
			17 Death
	5 Unplanned return to operating or delivery room on this admission		18 Subsequent visit to emergency room or outpatient department for complications or adverse results of this hospitalisation
	6 Surgical and other invasive procedures not meeting criteria for necessity and appropriateness. (a) Pathology report or preoperative diagnosis mismatch (b) Non-diagnostic tissue (c) No tissue (d) Other		19 Utilisation management variations from criteria for (a) Length of stay (c) Other (b) Resource utilisation
			20 Medical record review—physician (a) (c) (b) (d)
	7 Transfusion reactions, complications, and improper utilisation (a) Transfusion occasioned by atrogenic bleeding or anaemia (b) Transfusion not clinically indicated (c) Transfusion reaction		21 Medical record review—nursing (a) (c) (b) (d)
			22 Departmental or other problems
	8 Nosocomial (hospital acquired) infection		23 Patient or family dissatisfaction
	9 Antibiotic/drug utilisation which is unjustified, excessive, results in patient injury, or varies from approved criteria (a) (b)	Comments:	
	10 Cardiac or respiratory arrest or low Apgar score		
	11 Transfer from general care to special care unit (a) Complication (b) Utilisation problem		

*Reproduced with permission from *Health Services Management* 1989;**85**:178–81.

The care given to patients is objectively reviewed using: the screening criteria by specially trained screening staff, who are usually qualified nurses. When a case fits one or more of the screening criteria, the circumstances are carefully recorded, and the case is usually put forward for review by one of the clinician's peers. In some occurrence screening programmes the peer

TABLE II—Data collection form*

Hospital case no _____ Consultant code   *Inpatient/*day case
Date of admission _____ Date of discharge/____*Medical case/*surgical case
Transfer/death
Diagnosis on admission

		Nurses Kardex	Medical notes
1	Readmission (clinical complications after previous admission (Y/N) If Y, dates of original admission/s)		
2	Consent for operation (Y/N)		
3	Unplanned return to theatre (Y/N)		
4	Patient transfused (Y/N) If Y, transfusion reaction (Y/N)		
5	Hospital acquired infection (Y/N) If Y, type of infection		
6	Cardiac or respiratory arrest (Y/N)		
7	Hospital incident: Please tick (a) Accident—include data and incident (b) Intravenous catheter problems (c) Skin problems—for example, bedsores/rashes (d) Equipment failure (e) Others—for example, electric shock from hospital premises or equipment		
8	Transfer to special care unit (Y/N) If Y, give dates		
9	Transfer to other hospital (Y/N) If Y, date of transfer and name of hospital		
10	Death (Y/N)		
11	*Patient or *Family dissatisfaction (Y/N)		
12	Resuscitation category noted (Y/N) If Y, category		

		*Yes/*no	Date_____
13	Discharge note	*Yes/*no	Date_____
14	Discharge summary	*Yes/*no	Date_____
	Discharge summary: letter to doctor	*Yes/*no	Date _____
15	Property form signed for above admission	*Yes/*no	If no, previous admission *Yes/*no Date _____

*Reproduced with permission from *Health Services Management* 1989;**85**:178–81.

reviewer assesses the seriousness of the occurrence, considers what led to it, and makes a judgment about the standard of care that the patient received. If it merits it the particular case may be reviewed at an audit meeting, where trends in the number and type of cases, such as rates of wound infections, are also regularly examined. Occurrence screening provides a way of focusing on cases in which the standard of patient care may have been suboptimal and of systematically investigating and analysing the causes and contributory factors. The process of systematic investigation and analysis builds up a database of cases that can itself be analysed to identify trends or patterns or to compare clinical practice.

Occurrence screening is clearly well suited to multidisciplinary application—the criteria can relate to medical, nursing, paramedical, or non-clinical care—and appropriate review mechanisms for such criteria can be established. Indeed, because the technique can cover the whole of a patient's care it can reduce the duplication of effort inherent in a series of audit systems relating to individual professions and can identify concerns in quality assurance that cross professional boundaries and require joint professional action to resolve them. The ability of the technique to make use of simple generic criteria and more complex specialist criteria makes it highly flexible and adaptable to local circumstance.

Development of the technique

Occurrence screening was developed in California in the mid-1970s as a byproduct of a study of the potential level of claims about medical negligence.[5] That study tried to assess whether it would be financially feasible to introduce a no fault compensation scheme for victims of medical accidents by screening the care given to 20 000 inpatients at participating hospitals for "potentially compensable events." To do this a set of generalised criteria were designed to pick out cases for subsequent review by a team of clinicians and lawyers. The findings were unsurprising: compensating every patient who experienced such an event would be vastly more expensive than the existing costs of legal services, out of court settlements, and court awards. The researchers found, however, that the methods they had developed for the study could form the basis of a systematic and workable quality assurance tool. Subsequently one of the research team refined and improved the system and marketed it as the Medical Management Analysis

145

quality assurance and risk management system,[4] which is now used in over 200 hospitals in the United States.[3] Table I shows the set of 23 generic screening criteria recommended by Medical Management Analysis.

The use of occurrence screening systems as an important part of hospital quality assurance programmes, usually in tandem with rather than instead of other quality assurance techniques,[67] is now widespread in the United States. Occurrence screening is recommended by the American College of Surgeons and the American Society of Anesthesiology.[3] It is mandatory in all Department of Defence hospitals, and since July 1986 all professional review organisations have been using occurrence screening for reviewing records.[3] The suite of hospital wide clinical indicators recently developed by the Joint Commission for the Accreditation of Healthcare Organisations[89] is based on the topics highlighted as being significant in occurrence screening systems.[10]

Validity and reliability

Relatively few studies of the reliability and validity of occurrence screening as a measure of quality of care have been published. In 1986 a study of 426 patients with myocardial infarctions found a screening criteria measure both valid and reliable.[11] Yet in 1987 a study of 752 patients with a wide variety of diagnoses suggested that an occurrence screening had poor interobserver reliability.[12] More recently, an investigation of judgments concerning adverse events occurring during stay in hospital, which used multiple reviews of the records of 360 patients, found that such a review process can produce judgments which are both valid and reliable.[1314] There are many anecdotal accounts of the value and effectiveness of occurrence screening, but it is clear that its validity and reliability as a measure of the quality of care are far from proved.[15]

Occurrence screening in the United Kingdom

British hospitals have few existing locally managed mechanisms for routinely detecting, investigating, and analysing adverse patient occurrences. Those mechanisms that do exist, such as

146

accident reports, records of errors in medication, patient complaints, mortality and morbidity meetings, postmortem examinations, and so on, are rarely applied universally and often rely on the "self reporting" of adverse patient occurrences by those directly concerned with patient care. They usually exist in isolation and rarely form part of a coordinated quality assurance programme.

Pilot studies using occurrence screening techniques have been carried out at hospitals in Bath health authority (N Dixon, personal communication) and Brighton health authority.[16] Both studies have concentrated on identifying the applicability and practicability of the approach in the British setting. The Bath project is in progress, and major trials in the acute setting are now being planned at the Royal Sussex County Hospital in Brighton and in the acute unit of Bromley health authority.[17]

Pilot study

In 1988 a pilot study of 250 patients' medical records was carried out at Hove General Hospital.[16] The intention was to establish whether an occurrence screening measure could be adapted for use in a British acute hospital, to ascertain the feasibility of using patients' medical records as the information source for screening, and to identify any unforeseen difficulties with the method. A set of 11 generic criteria were selected for use in the pilot study, and their definitions were translated into English (rather than American) terminology. Four additional criteria were developed locally. Table II shows the criteria used. The screening of patient records against these criteria was carried out by an experienced medical administrator without medical or nursing training. A sample of her screening was then checked by a doctor, who found no errors in her work and judged that in those instances in which she had been unsure a qualified nurse would have been able to be more certain. The screener's time was used most efficiently by screening notes soon after discharge. This made the notes easier to locate and simplified the task of identifying what information in the notes related to the most recent admission. Under these circumstances over 90% of cases took less than 10 minutes each to screen.

The results of screening in the pilot study indicate the rates of adverse patient occurrences that might be encountered in a larger trial. It was found that 22% of patients had at least one adverse patient occurrence during their stay (studies in the United States

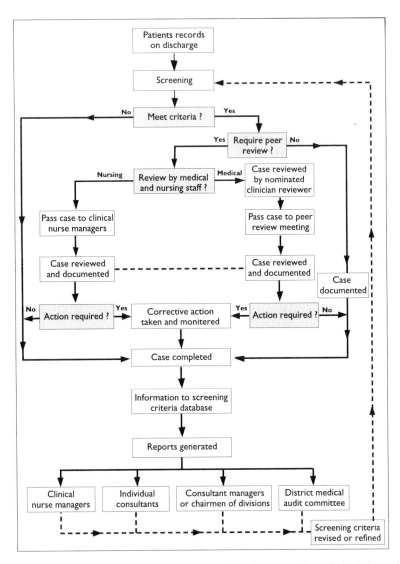

suggest that around 18–20% of patients have an adverse patient occurrence while in hospital[18]). The commonest occurrence (experienced by a tenth of all patients in the study) was a hospital acquired infection. Four per cent of patients, however, had incomplete operation consent forms, 2% had a cardiac or respiratory arrest, 3% had problems related to intravenous cannulas or catheters, and 1% had a slip or fall during their stay.[16]

It proved difficult to apply some of the criteria, such as those relating to evidence of patient or family dissatisfaction and to the standard of discharge documentation, solely on the basis of the information in the patient's medical records. The results of the pilot study were, however, largely encouraging and confirmed that the method could be applied practically in a British hospital.

Occurrence screening project

In mid-1989 Brighton health authority and CASPE Research were awarded finance from the Department of Health's central fund for medical audit to test whether occurrence screening could form the basis of a hospital wide approach to medical audit at the district's main acute services site, the Royal Sussex County Hospital, which has over 22 000 discharges and deaths per year. With the participation of consultant medical staff and joint medical and managerial leadership, a three year project plan was designed. The project has four main aims. Firstly, to investigate the reliability and validity of occurrence screening as a measure of quality of hospital care. Secondly, to foster the development of peer review mechanisms among medical and nursing staff so that the information gathered by screening can be appropriately analysed and investigated; in the process it is planned to develop accurate, timely, and comprehensible formats for reporting screening information to clinicians. Thirdly, to establish whether a combination of peer review mechanisms and meaningful reports facilitate changes in clinical practice if these prove to be necessary. Finally, to establish benchmarks for the costs associated with the use of occurrence screening so that its cost effectiveness can be clearly identified. Because of the differences in organisational structure and professional practice in hospitals in the United States and Britain the American model for peer review is not wholly suited to a British setting, and we plan to use a revised model (figure).

In parallel with the Brighton project, a cooperative commercial development of an occurrence screening system is in progress in the acute unit of Bromley health authority, sponsored by South

East Thames Regional Health Authority. The two project teams intend to meet regularly and pool experience and skill.

Conclusions

Experience in the United States and initial research in Britain suggest that occurrence screening systems may provide a highly effective approach to audit that can accommodate the requirements of a wide variety of medical specialties. Though such systems are clearly limited in their remit and take little account of important issues such as the appropriateness of care or its opportunity costs, it is evident that they can make a major contribution to maintenance and improvement of overall standards of care for hospital patients. In the light of the white paper *Working for Patients*[19] and the statement in its associated working paper that all doctors (not just all consultants) should be involved in medical audit by April 1991, occurrence screening may prove highly relevant to the fast changing needs of the NHS.

1 Stevens G, Wickings I, Bennett J. Medical quality assurance: research in Brighton health authority. *International Journal of Healthcare Quality Assurance* 1988;1:5–11.
2 Bowden D, Williams G, Stevens G. Medical quality assurance in Brighton—can American translate into English? In: Moores B, ed. *Are they being served?* Oxford: Philip Allan, 1986:104–14.
3 Carlow D. Occurrence screening can improve QA programs. *Dimens Health Serv* 1988;65:20–2.
4 Craddick JW. The medical management analysis system—a professional liability warning system. *QRB* 1979;5:2–8.
5 California Medical Association and California Hospital Association. *Report on the medical insurance feasibility study*. San Francisco: Sutter Publications, 1977.
6 Walczak R. Occurrence screening: is it worth it? *Quality, Risk and Cost Advisor* 1984;1:1–7.
7 Burmeister RW. Occurrence screening: only the means to an end. *Quality, Risk and Cost Advisor* 1986;2:5–6.
8 Robinson ML. Sneak preview: JCAHO's quality indicators. *Hospitals* 1988;62:38–43.
9 Shaw CD. Clinical outcome indicators. *Health Trends* 1988;21:37–40.
10 Hopkins J. QA methodologies. *Quality, Risk and Cost Advisor* 1989;5:7.
11 Panniers TL, Newlander J. The adverse patient occurrences inventory: validity, reliability and implications. *QRB* 1986;12:311–5.
12 Schumacher DN, Parker B, Kofie V, *et al*. Severity of illness index and the adverse patient occurrence index: a reliability study and policy implications. *Med Care* 1987;25:695–704.
13 Brennan TA, Localio RJ, Laird NL. Reliability and validity of judgments concerning adverse events suffered by hospitalised patients. *Med Care* 1989;27:1148–58.
14 Brennan TA, Localio RJ, Leape LL, *et al*. Identification of adverse events occurring during hospitalisation. *Ann Intern Med* 1990;112:221–6.
15 Van Cleave EF. Uses of risk adjusted outcomes in quality assurance monitoring. In: Spath PL, ed. *Innovations in healthcare quality management*. Chicago: American Hospital Publishing, 1989:1–9.
16 Stevens G, Bennett J. Clinical audit—occurrence screening for quality assurance. *Health Services Management* 1989;85:178–81.
17 South East Thames Regional Health Authority. *Briefing: new medical audit process for Britain*. Bexhill: SETRHA, 1989.

18 Craddick JW, Bader B. *Medical management analysis: a systematic approach to quality assurance and risk management*. Auburn, California: Joyce W Craddick, 1983:7.
19 Secretaries of State for Health, Wales, Northern Ireland, and Scotland. *Working for patients*. London: HMSO, 1989(Cm555).

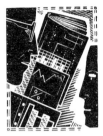

Surveys of patient satisfaction: I—Important general considerations

RAY FITZPATRICK

Why conduct a survey?

Discussions about how the quality of health care should be measured increasingly include patient satisfaction as one of the important dimensions.[1][2] However, a single explanation of why surveys of patients' views have suddenly become such a visible and regular aspect of the NHS would probably not cite the impact of scientific arguments about the evaluation of health services but the far more influential NHS Management Inquiry. The inquiry crisply and emphatically condemned the failure of the NHS to use the well established techniques of market research to elicit the views and experiences of its users.[3] The proliferation of surveys that immediately followed that report was largely managerially led and focused on subjects that managers may have felt more competent or confident to tackle, such as the quality of catering and physical amenities provided for inpatients or the accessibility of health care facilities.

Subsequently, important statements from professional bodies argued along similar lines to those of the government's white paper *Working for Patients*[4] by underlining the wider contribution of patients' views to assessing quality of care in hospitals and primary care.[5][6] It will be unlikely, if these recommendations are heeded, that surveys will continue to concentrate narrowly on so called "hotel" aspects of health care, such as catering. The patient's views will increasingly be sought on such matters as information needs; interpersonal and organisational aspects of care; and, indeed, the value of medical treatments.

There are three reasons besides external pressures from governments, professional bodies, and health authorities why health professionals should take patient satisfaction seriously as a measurement (box). Firstly, there is convincing evidence that satisfaction is an important outcome measure. It may be a predictor of whether patients follow their recommended treatments,[7] and is related to whether patients reattend for treatment[8] and change their provider of health care.[9] Evidence has also begun to emerge that satisfaction is related to improvements in health status.[10 11] Secondly, patient satisfaction is an increasingly useful measure in assessing consultations and patterns of communication (such as the success of giving information, of involving the patient in decisions about care, and of reassurance).[12] Thirdly, patient feedback can be used systematically to choose between alternative methods of organising or providing health care (such as length of consultation or arrangements for out of hours care).[13]

Patient satisfaction as measure of health care

- An important outcome measure
- Useful in assessing consultations and patterns of communication
- Used systematically, feedback enables choice between alternatives in organising or providing health care

---

Health professionals remain largely unfamiliar with methods of measurement derived from survey research. This paper considers some of the potential problems and strategic questions involved in surveys of patient satisfaction. A subsequent article will examine some of the main considerations involved in designing, conducting, and analysing a survey of patients' views.

Why not to conduct a survey

The time, resources, and staff required to design, conduct, and analyse a survey are invariably underestimated. Given that various costs are associated with even the most modest survey, alternative

153

methods of obtaining the desired information or goal should always be seriously considered. For example, in general terms we already know much about many of the matters most commonly associated with patient dissatisfaction.[14] With regard to hospital care, well established complaints would include waiting for an outpatient appointment or admission, waiting at clinics, and inadequate or poor information at all stages and about most matters of concern to the patient. In primary care patients' criticisms may focus on problems of access such as appointment systems and out of hours care, problems of rapport with the doctor and, again, limitations in communication between health professional and patient. Thus it may be sufficient to review the growing number of publications. Furthermore, if the object of the survey is to sensitise staff to the patient's point of view there are numerous alternative possibilities—from establishing patient participation groups through tape recording and playing back to staff individual patients' accounts of their experiences—that may be better than a survey. A survey should be used to answer a question, and the more precisely that question is formulated, the more successful the survey is likely to prove. The question need not be in the form of a hypothesis. Surveys are frequently descriptive in intent, to ascertain which aspects of care are related to the highest and lowest levels of satisfaction in a given patient group. However, measures of people's perceptions and views are increasingly shown to have measurement properties as robust in terms of reliability and reproducibility as physiological and other conventional medical measures.[15] It is then appropriate to ask more specific questions by means of measures of satisfaction, particularly in evaluating health care.

Negative assumptions about surveys of patient satisfaction

- Uncover widespread and general dissatisfaction
- Answers are ill considered or whimsical
- Misjudgments arising from patients' reliance on perceptions based on surrogate indicators (halo effect)

Some prejudices about patient surveys

It is worth while confronting several negative assumptions that may exist about the value of surveys of patient satisfaction (box).

One unspoken anxiety may be that they will uncover widespread and general dissatisfaction, which will prove undermining to all concerned. However, health professionals seem to estimate greater levels of dissatisfaction in their patients than surveys disclose.[16] Virtually all surveys indicate only a few patients who express negative views about any particular issue. Indeed, one of the greatest single problems in this type of work is the lack of variability in results; typically, at least 80% of respondents express satisfaction for any given question. One reason is the reluctance of many patients in the NHS to express critical comments about their health care.[17]

A more commonly expressed reservation is that answers given to surveys of satisfaction will reflect essentially ill considered, whimsical, or unstable thoughts and feelings, especially given the emotional and fluctuating nature of many episodes of illness. A variant of this concern is the argument that because of the technical complexity of so many aspects of health care patients are not competent to make sensible judgments about much of the care that they receive. In particular, patients might be thought to depend for their judgments on factors that from a health professional's viewpoint are potentially misleading. Some research evidence can be cited to fuel such anxieties. One study suggested that patients' views about the technical skills and medical competence of their personal doctors as expressed in a survey were largely determined by their perceptions of quite different qualities of the doctor—the extent of friendly and reassuring interpersonal manners.[18] Psychologists have long recognised the importance of such "halo effects" in attitudinal surveys, whereby single striking impressions of another person colour and shape all other judgments made about them.

However, the more specific and well designed the questionnaire, the clearer it is that patients do not respond in terms of global reactions, and they may form quite distinct views about different aspects of a single episode of a health care consultation. Moreover, as with other fields of survey research and measurement of attitude, reservations such as those expressed above have to be taken account of by examining the reliability and validity of questionnaires.

Reliability is concerned with the extent to which a questionnaire produces the same results on separate occasions of use. Clearly, examining such features is not easy, given that there may be low agreement between two administrations of a questionnaire, which may be due to real changes in patients' views. Remarkably few studies have examined what is formally known as the "test-retest" reliability of questionnaires of patient satisfaction, but the results have been encouraging.[19] An alternative approach is by examining "internal reliability." One common form of this is "split half" reliability, which examines the extent of agreement between the halves of a questionnaire or section of a questionnaire considered to be measuring a particular dimension of satisfaction. Again, results of such examinations are satisfactory.[20]

Validity is much more difficult to examine and, compared with reliability, is beyond the means of most simple surveys to evaluate in any real sense. This is because validity of a questionnaire is the requirement for it to measure what it claims to measure, and it is difficult to imagine any ultimate gold standard against which to assess a questionnaire of satisfaction. However, some elaborate studies showed that such questionnaires can relate to other measures in theoretically expected ways (so called "construct validity"). Patients' views about consultations as expressed in questionnaires correlate with independent measures of doctors' interpersonal skills,[21] communication styles,[22] and technical proficiency.[23]

Strategic considerations

Some strategic issues of choice confront investigators about to conduct a survey. Firstly, it is clear that far from having one global reaction to their health care that may be captured in an overall question about their satisfaction, patients have distinct and differentiated views that may, in principle, be captured by a questionnaire. One of the most elaborate investigations was able to show that patients held distinct views on at least four broad dimensions of their health care: the doctor's conduct, availability of care, continuity and convenience, and financial accessibility.[24] However, a full list of dimensions in terms of which patients' views have been examined would be much larger (box). The investigator therefore needs to consider which aspects are relevant to the research question. Studies have been much more likely to include dimensions such as humaneness and information-giving whereas, surprisingly, patients' views on outcomes have been neglected.[25]

Different dimensions of patient satisfaction

- Humaneness
- Informativeness
- Overall quality
- Competence
- Bureaucracy
- Access

- Cost
- Facilities
- Outcome
- Continuity
- Attention to psychosocial problems

A second broad consideration is whether to gather information by means of a self completed questionnaire or by interview, and this is likely to be particularly influenced by resources. The balance sheet of advantages between the two methods (box) gives some indication of the different considerations relevant to a decision. It is often argued that an interview will always "outperform" a questionnaire in obtaining sensitive information accurately. However, there is no reason to believe that a carefully developed and well piloted self completed questionnaire should be quite such a second best choice as the list suggests.

A final aspect that is rarely considered at the time of embarking on a study is how the results are to be disseminated and ultimately acted on. Yet one of the key lessons from the managerial phase of activity in the research on patient satisfaction in the NHS must surely be the problems that arise from lack of attention given to

---

Advantages of self completed versus interview questionnaires

Interview	*Self completed*
Sensitivity to patients' concerns	Standardisation of items
Flexibility in covering topics	No "interviewer bias"
Rapport	Anonymity
Clarification of ambiguities of items or of reasons for views	Low cost of data gathering
Respondent adherence More scope to follow up non-respondents	Less need for trained staff

---

this issue.[26] Conducting a survey requires motivation and involvement by many staff, as well as the vital contributions of patients. Yet all too commonly reports of surveys are filed away without apparently having had any purpose or consequences, resulting in widespread disillusionment with the exercise. As much care is therefore needed in deciding how surveys are to be integrated into the continuous process of providing and improving care as in considering the scientific issues of survey design.

1 Maxwell R. Quality assessment in health. *BMJ* 1984;**288**:1470–2.
2 Hopkins A, Costain D, eds. *Measuring the outcomes of medical care*. London: Royal College of Physicians and King's Fund Centre, 1990.
3 Department of Health and Social Security. *NHS management inquiry. Report*. London: DHSS, 1983.
4 Secretaries of State for Health, Wales, Northern Ireland, and Scotland. *Working for patients*. London: HMSO, 1989. (Cm 555.)
5 Royal College of General Practitioners. *Quality in general practice*. London: RCGP, 1985. (Policy statement No 2.)
6 Hopkins A. *Measuring the quality of medical care*. London: Royal College of Physicians, 1990.
7 Kincey J, Bradshaw P, Ley P. Patients' satisfaction and reported acceptance of advice in general practice. *J R Coll Gen Pract* 1975;**25**:558–66.
8 Roghmann K, Hengst A, Zastowny T. Satisfaction with medical care: its measurement and relation to utilisation. *Med Care* 1979;**17**:461–77.
9 Weiss B, Senf J. Patient satisfaction survey instrument for use in health maintenance organisation. *Med Care* 1990;**28**:434–45.
10 Fitzpatrick R, Hopkins A, Harvard-Watts O. Social dimensions of healing: a longitudinal study of outcomes of medical management of headaches. *Soc Sci Med* 1983;**17**:501–10.
11 Fitzpatrick R, Bury M, Frank A, Donnelly T. Problems in the assessment of outcome in a back pain clinic. *International Rehabilitation Studies* 1987;**9**:161–5.
12 Savage R, Armstrong D. Effect of a general practitioner's consulting style on patients' satisfaction: a controlled study. *BMJ* 1990;**301**:968–70.
13 Bollam M, McCarthy M, Modell M. Patients' assessments of out of hours care in general practice. *BMJ* 1988;**296**:829–32.
14 Fitzpatrick R. Satisfaction with health care. In: Fitzpatrick R, Hinton J, Newman S, Scambler G, Thompson J, eds. *The experience of illness*. London: Tavistock, 1984:154–78.
15 Feinstein A. Clinical biostatistics, XLI. Hard science, soft data, and the challenges of choosing clinical variables in research. *Clin Pharmacol Ther* 1977;**22**:485–98.
16 Rashid A, Forman W, Jagger C, Mann R. Consultations in general practice: a comparison of patients' and doctors' satisfaction. *BMJ* 1990;**299**:1015–6.
17 Fitzpatrick R, Hopkins A. Problems in the conceptual framework of patient satisfaction research. *Sociology of Health and Illness* 1983;**5**:297–311.
18 Sira ZB. Affective and instrumental components in the physician-patient relationship. *J Health Soc Behav* 1980;**21**:170–80.
19 Korsch B, Gozzi E, Francis V. Gaps in doctor-patient communications. 1. Doctor-patient interaction and patient satisfaction. *Pediatrics* 1968;**42**:855–71.
20 Baker R. Development of a questionnaire to assess patients' satisfaction with consultations in general practice. *British Journal of General Practice* 1990;**40**:487–90.
21 DiMatteo R, Taranta A, Fiedman H, Prince L. Predicting patient satisfaction from physicians' nonverbal communication skills. *Med Care* 1980;**18**:376–87.
22 Stiles W, Putnam S, Wolf M, James S. Interaction exchange structure and patient satisfaction with medical interviews. *Med Care* 1979;**17**:667–81.
23 Roter D, Hall J, Katz N. Relations between physicians' behaviors and analogue patients' satisfaction, recall and impressions. *Med Care* 1987;**25**:437–51.

24 Ware J, Snyder M. Dimensions of patient attitudes regarding doctors and medical care services. *Med Care* 1975;**13**:669–79.

25 Hall J, Dorman M. What patients like about their medical care and how often they are asked: a meta-analysis of the satisfaction literature. *Soc Sci Med* 1988;**27**:935–40.

26 Dixon P, Carr-Hill R. *The NHS and its customers: III. Customer feedback surveys—a review of current practice.* York: Centre for Health Economics, University of York, 1989.

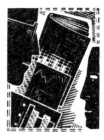

Surveys of patient satisfaction: II—Designing a questionnaire and conducting a survey

RAY FITZPATRICK

This article considers some of the basic issues in designing a survey of patient satisfaction, particularly developing or selecting a questionnaire and conducting and analysing a survey. A few instruments have been developed by research teams for widespread use in the NHS. Examples include a hospital patient questionnaire developed by Clinical Accountability, Service Planning, and Evaluation (CASPE)[1]; a questionnaire to measure satisfaction with consultations developed for use in general practice[2]; and a questionnaire to measure satisfaction with breast screening.[3] Investigators can use such instruments knowing that some basic properties such as reliability and acceptability will have already been established (although it is always wise to examine carefully the published details of such developmental work). Another advantage may be that there may be other data with which their own eventual results can be directly compared. However, most surveys of patients' views tend to be based on a questionnaire that the investigators have developed themselves.

Questionnaires of patient satisfaction take one of two forms: they may be either episode specific or more general in terms of the focus of the questions. Those that are episode specific tend to include questionnaire items such as, "Did the doctor give you a clear enough explanation of what was wrong with you?" whereas a more general focus would be provided by, "Does your doctor give you sufficiently clear explanations of what is wrong with you?". The choice will depend partly on the type of health care setting and partly on the research question. A recent meta-analysis of studies of patient satisfaction concluded that questionnaires with more episode specific content tend to produce more uniformly favourable responses from patients compared with somewhat more negative views elicited by means of generally worded questions.[4] When patients are asked for their views about health care in general terms, it is suggested that they draw on more negative stereotypes about health care facilities whereas in surveys focused on specific episodes they may have an optimistic bias to assume that their own experience is better than that of others. The meta-analysis was heavily dependent on American surveys, and it is by no means clear that the same differences between methods would occur in Great Britain. The argument for episode specific questionnaire items is that they should reflect more accurately individuals' actual experiences. One study that did directly compare general questions with specific questions for a single sample of patients found that the specific questions resulted in more variation in answers.[5]

A second broad choice of approach is between questions which directly ask about level of satisfaction ("How satisfied were you with . . .?") compared with indirect approaches in which satisfaction is inferred from the choice of answer. For example, a positive answer to, "Did the doctor answer all of the questions about your problem?" would be interpreted as a satisfied response. There are no established advantages to either approach.

As was argued in my previous article[6] it is clear that patient satisfaction is multidimensional. As a result questionnaires increasingly tend to ask more specific and focused questions rather than ask for global judgments of how satisfied the person is. The more clearly focused each question, the easier it is to compare satisfaction with the different elements of care.

The form of answers offered to the respondent in the questionnaires varies. The simplest form of response is "yes" or "no." The advantages of simplicity of this format are, according to many survey analysts, outweighed by the fact that most respondents will give the favourable answer to any item about health care. This is a major problem given the overall need to maximise the variability of responses in any survey. Therefore most survey questionnaires now favour more than two alternative responses per question (for example, respondents select from four or five possible answers in a range from "very satisfied" through to "very dissatisfied"). The respondent is given a greater opportunity to express the precise nature of his or her view. Moreover, the reliability of items increases as the number of response alternatives increases.[7] In practice the gain in precision or reliability of increasing the possible answers beyond seven is minimal, and generally five response categories are used.[7]

More advanced questionnaires tend to be developed from more general principles of attitude measurement. In particular, several different items may be asked about one issue in the form of a Likert scale of items, each of which typically has five responses from "strongly agree" to "strongly disagree," which are given a numerical score (box). The summed score of all the items is taken to represent the person's underlying view or attitude. Again, psychometric analysis has shown that Likert summed scales are more reliable than individual items.[8] The second box shows an example of such a scale taken from a study of patient satisfaction among chronically ill patients.[9] The third item also illustrates a conventional wisdom of questionnaire design: that "response acquiescence"—the tendency to agree rather than to disagree—should be allowed for by some items with reversed wording and the scoring appropriately reversed. The assumption that several items all contribute to the measurement of a single underlying view or attitude is something that has to be checked statistically on a pilot sample before it can be properly used in a scale. Techniques such as factor analysis are used for this purpose.

Examples of Likert scale of questionnaire items

"The doctor gave me a helpful explanation of what was wrong with me"
5 = strongly agree, 4 = agree, 3 = uncertain, 2 = disagree, 1 = strongly disagree

---

There are more general, commonsense considerations in the design of a questionnaire. If it is for self completion the questionnaire needs to be easy to follow and attractively set out. It is most important to include a simple, clear statement of the purpose and

> Summed scale of satisfaction among chronically ill patients
>
> (1) I am in better health now because of the care I received there
> (2) The doctors did as much as could be expected to help me get well
> (3) Some of the things the doctor did were not very helpful
> (4) The doctors helped me feel a lot better
> Each item scored from 5 (strongly agree) to 1 (strongly disagree), except item 3 in which scoring is reversed. Total range of scores from 4 to 20

use of the questionnaire and explanations of why the person has been selected, how the questionnaire is to be completed, and what the person is to do with it after its completion.

Other items to be included

It is routine in survey research to include what are commonly referred to as "background variables"—that is, social and demographic variables. They have particular importance in research of patient satisfaction because variables such as age, sex, education, social class, and marital status may all exert as strong an influence on levels of satisfaction as any direct effect of health services. Only age seems consistently to be related to satisfaction, with younger respondents expressing less positive satisfaction. It is often difficult to clarify whether the relation between such variables and satisfaction is due to differences in expectations and readiness to express negative views or actual differences in the quality of health care received.[10] Now that reliable and brief social survey instruments exist to measure health status,[11] and given the frequently observed relation between health status and patient satisfaction,[12] a simple measure of health status might also be included.

Piloting a questionnaire

It is essential that a questionnaire be piloted on a sample of respondents before the full survey. This will allow several potential problems to be predicted. Firstly, the clarity and acceptability of questionnaire items can be examined. Also, if respondents are given space for open ended comments additional items or issues not included in the first draft of a questionnaire may emerge. In addition, the variability of answers may be checked. The survey will not be particularly informative if the final version of the questionnaire includes too many items that produce uniform responses. It may even pay to have a phase of prepilot open ended, exploratory interviewing, in which the full range and dimensions of patients' views are assessed, before proceeding to the fixed, closed questionnaire items of the pilot. Other aspects of the survey such as method of explanation and presentational aspects of the questionnaire may also be tested at this stage, and this is also the best opportunity, if possible, to examine formal properties of a questionnaire, such as reliability.

Survey sample

It is important to be clear about the population whose views are relevant in any particular survey. For example, in one survey only the views and attitudes of patients who have actually attended and used a particular clinic may be wanted. For a different kind of inquiry including patients who have not recently attended the facility may be vitally important; their views may be appreciably different from those of the attenders.

Having decided on the relevant population, survey researchers then face the decision whether to conduct a *census* of every individual in the population or to obtain the views of a *sample*, in which case the aim is to construct a sample that can represent the entire population while avoiding the many costs that might be expected from gathering every person's views, as in a census. In addition to considerations of cost, statisticians argue that for most purposes a sample is probably superior to a census because the potential biases entailed in trying but failing to include all individuals in a census may be more effectively controlled in a smaller scale sampling procedure. Should investigators opt for a sample, several further decisions follow. Either they may conduct a *random sample* or some alternative to the random sample such as *quota sampling*. A random sample is not exactly that. Rather than respondents being chosen haphazardly or without pattern, it requires a process whereby each member of a population is given an equal chance of falling into the sample. Formal random sampling generally requires recourse to a table of random numbers. A more practical variant of random sampling that is unlikely to be seriously flawed is *systematic sampling*, whereby, for example, every tenth patient is selected. This would be a problem only if the systematic sample had something in common, for example, if it comprised patients given shorter consultation times by the appointments system.

A somewhat different approach, used in public opinion polls, is the *quota sample*, in which the investigators decide that three or four variables are potentially important to respondents' views— commonly these might include age, sex, and social class. The objective is to construct a sample representative of the population with regard to these variables. A predetermined number of men and women and young and old respondents would be obtained; with other variables the sample would be haphazard and based on availability. Whatever method is adopted, any survey will be more convincing if every reasonable effort has been made to recruit initial non-respondents, by follow up. Further advice is now readily available on issues of sampling in surveys of patient satisfaction.[13]

Conduct of survey

Two broad principles need to be adhered to as far as possible, the anonymity and confidentiality of the respondent's answers and the neutrality of the person gathering the data. Both are primarily designed to maximise the candid expression of views. The principle of anonymity is completely achieved if no method of identifying respondents is used, but some technique such as identification by code numbers is needed if follow up of non-respondents is to be achieved. Statements of confidentiality require a simple explanation of how information is to be processed and analysed. Many surveys attempt to guarantee the neutrality of the person gathering the data by involving research institutes or academic groups, which are less closely identified with health care providers, in collecting and analysing the data, but this may not always be feasible. It would be reasonable to assume that the setting in which the respondents express their views would influence results, so that, for example, they were more frank in the privacy of their own homes. However, the one systematic analysis of the effect of setting failed to find any evidence to support such views.[4]

Analysis

Details about analysis are beyond the scope of this article, but one general point can be emphasised. Sensible analysis and interpretation of a survey of patient satisfaction will require at least two kinds of manipulation of variables, which means that a computer, and most probably a statistical package such as the statistical package for the social sciences (SPSS) or SAS will be highly desirable. These requirements obviously need to be anticipated from the outset. The two kinds of manipulation of variables that are almost inevitable are (*a*) combining single satisfaction items into summed scales and (*b*) subgroup analysis. The value of summed scales has been explained in the context of reliability. The need for subgroup analysis is a direct consequence of the effects that demographic, social, and other "background" variables may have on satisfaction. Suppose, for example, that a significant difference in satisfaction was found between two group practices, two wards, or two doctors. Before taking the result seriously as evidence that some aspect of the service was responsible for the difference, it would be essential to establish that it was not an artefact of other differences between the two groups of patients, such as in age or health status. This can be examined only by manipulating the data to "control" for possible confounding effects.

Methods of survey sampling

- Random sampling
- Systematic sampling
- Quota sampling

Subgroup analysis has another role in studies of patient satisfaction and, indeed, in survey analysis more generally. Important relations may emerge only from such analysis. To take two simple examples, in a randomised trial of fee for service care compared with enrolment into a health maintenance organisation differences in satisfaction between the two groups of patients were clearest among those with higher incomes but poorer health status.[14] In a study of satisfaction with primary care among elderly people satisfaction was related to whether the doctor showed personal interest in the patient only among those of poorer health status.[15] The survey makes its greatest contribution to knowledge when relations between variables are clarified and "specified" in this way, and methods of doing this have been clearly described.[16] By going beyond the basic reporting of proportions of individuals satisfied with this or that aspect of care, investigators contribute not only to a more accurate understanding of the specific topic covered in the survey but also to the broader questions of how patients respond to and evaluate their health care.

1 Green J. On the receiving end. *Health Services Journal* 1988;**98**:880–2.
2 Baker R. Development of a questionnaire to assess patients' satisfaction with consultations in general practice. *British Journal of General Practice* 1990;**40**:487–90.
3 Eardley A, Lancaster G, Elkind A. Made to measure survey. *Health Services Journal* 1990;**100**:1773.
4 Hall J, Dornan M. Meta-analysis of satisfaction with medical care: description of research domain and analysis of overall satisfaction levels. *Soc Sci Med* 1988;**27**:637–44.
5 Pascoe G, Attkinson C. The Evaluation Ranking Scale: a new methodology for assessing satisfaction. *Evaluation and Program Planning* 1983;**6**:335–47.
6 Fitzpatrick R. Surveys of patient satisfaction: I—Important general considerations. *BMJ* 1991;**302**:887–9.
7 Nunnally J. *Psychometric theory*. New York: McGraw Hill, 1967.
8 Oppenheim A. *Questionnaire design and attitude measurement*. London: Heinemann, 1966.
9 Linn L, Greenfield S. Patient suffering and patient satisfaction among the chronically ill. *Med Care* 1982;**20**:425–31.
10 Fitzpatrick R. Satisfaction with health care. In: Fitzpatrick R, Hinton J, Newman S, Scambler G, Thompson J, eds. *The experience of illness*. London: Tavistock, 1984:154–78.
11 Fallowfield L. *The quality of life: the missing measurement in health care*. London: Souvenir Press, 1990.
12 Hall J, Feldstein M, Fretwell M, *et al*. Older patients' health status and satisfaction with medical care in an HMO population. *Med Care* 1990;**28**:261–70.
13 Dixon P, Carr-Hill R. *The NHS and its customers: II. Customer feedback surveys—an introduction to survey methods*. York: Centre for Health Economics, University of York, 1989.
14 Davies A, Ware J, Brook R, Peterson J, Newhouse J. Consumer acceptance of prepaid and fee for service medical care: results from a randomised controlled trial. *Health Serv Res* 1986;**21**:429–52.
15 Snider E. The elderly and their doctors. *Soc Sci Med* 1980;**14A**:527–31.
16 Marsh C. *The survey method*. London: Allen and Unwin, 1982.

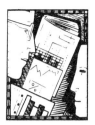

LEARNING AND AUDIT

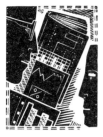

Educational aspects
of medical audit

G F BATSTONE

Medical Audit: Working Paper 6[1] does not couch medical audit activities in an educational environment. The Royal College of Physicians and Royal College of Surgeons, however, have highlighted the educational aspects of medical audit, stating that "education is the most useful product of audit"[2] and that audit "is an important educational process for both seniors and juniors."[3] Kenneth Clarke in a speech on 10 July stated that in his view, "Medical audit is about quality assurance in clinical work. As it entails a measurement of performance it must be a key part of continuing professional education." This echoes the theme of the report of the Alment Committee: "In our view it is a necessary part of a doctor's professional responsibility to assess his work regularly in association with his colleagues,"[4] although in medical audit such reviews are considered educational. The approach of peer review of practice creates a "sympathetic environment" for medical audit.

This paper aims at highlighting the educational aspects of audit and the framework required to exploit them and at considering the nature of education and of audit.

Educational aspects

Medical audit works at two levels: firstly, through individual self assessment and professional development, and, secondly, through review of performance by the clinical team, leading to enhancement of the quality of activity of that team. Thus audit may be regarded as a process leading to improved clinical care by mechanisms which may be educational or operational, or both. The educational strengths of audit are:

- Small group work, which is effective in modifying attitudes and management of clinical conditions
- Critical review of current practice, which encourages learning about new techniques and treatments and when to use them
- Review of current practice, leading to reinforcement of agreed procedures and thus making teaching junior doctors more explicit and practice based
- Observation of practice, which may indicate gaps in knowledge and skills for which appropriate educational programmes may be developed.

Audit also discloses operational features that require modification to enhance quality of patient care, which may include problems associated with communication, motivation, explicitness of procedures, weakness of structure or organisation of clinical work, or inappropriate use of resources. To overcome these problems doctors require skills for counselling those who seem poorly motivated; for use of briefing systems to ensure that members of the clinical team are aware of developments; for reviews of procedures to ensure that these are up to date and well understood; for enhancement of structures to make them efficient; and for making judgments on priorities for use of resources. These skills are largely parallel to management approaches such as "action centred leadership"[5] and are very different from many "management courses" to which senior registrars and consultants are subjected. Here, therefore, is another educational and training area that requires attention if audit is to be successful in effecting changes that improve patient care.

Organisational aspects

The white paper indicates the need for a clearly defined organisational framework for audit, led by a senior clinician, who will require appropriate training. As each district hospital and family practitioner committee sets up audit advisory committees it will be essential for them to recognise the need to link with educational organisations at district level. Some districts have recognised this requirement by using the district medical education committee[6] as their audit advisory committee. Most districts have a district medical education committee (according to a postal survey by the National Association of Clinical Tutors with a 40% response rate,

82% of postgraduate centres had working committees with a further 10% planned), and these comprise clinical tutors and college tutors with the director of public health and additional general practice representatives. Such a body can plan educational programmes for individual doctors or clinical teams to overcome deficiencies in knowledge and skills identified by audit. It is unreasonable to expect any other district body to be able to help in developing reading plans, literature reviews, computer and video packages, specific training courses, and even secondment.

Audit in educational programmes

Most doctors in training or continuing medical education will need help with setting standards, techniques for monitoring performance against these standards, and determining the source of any apparent shortfall in the service studied. Newcomers to audit will require help in selecting appropriate topics with achievable outcomes in order to maintain their enthusiasm. Also, development of training in management techniques to improve the effectiveness and efficiency of clinical teams will be required if audit is to be central to decision making processes.

Audit also has a role in continuing medical education. In medical training Harden recommended the concept of "task based learning" to link clinical experiences of cases with theoretical information to provide a learning environment.[7] Within continuing medical education audit topics may be used in a programme of journal clubs, case discussions, and lectures by external experts to link current clinical experience, knowledge, and skills with new information to promote learning that changes behaviour. Such a curriculum requires careful planning and much skill to be effective.

Nature of education and audit

Education has been defined variously as: (*a*) the passing on of a cultural heritage; (*b*) the initiation into worthwhile fashions of behaviour; and (*c*) the fostering of an individual's growth, and audit has strong links with the last two statements. For adult education to be successful learning tasks should be used that build on earlier learning and there should be feedback on development of skills, time for reflection by learners on their approaches, and a

173

choice of approaches for acquiring new skills and knowledge.[8] The reflective aspects of professional knowledge and action as explored by Schon[9] is a necessary step in turning experience into learning. Another important aspect of the "elaborated learner" emphasises the ability to transfer knowledge to fresh circumstances. These factors are linked in the learning cycle described by Kolb (fig 1).[10] The cycle begins with observation of and reflection on current practice to ascertain the principles for care, which are then applied in new environments. This cycle is rather different from the audit cycle,[2] which starts by setting standards and then by observation assesses conformity with them. The critical part is to determine the cause of any deficiency and then to implement changes to rectify the situation (fig 2).

Resolution of the apparent differences between these two cycles has been attempted.[11] One difficulty with the audit cycle is the

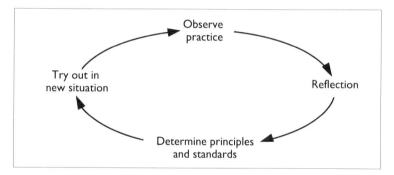

FIG 1—Learning cycle (after Kolb[10])

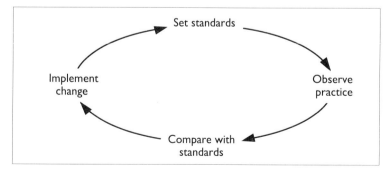

FIG 2—Audit cycle (after Royal College of Physicians)

setting of standards, and for many this is best achieved by observing practice and reflecting on its aims. This process is often triggered by an unexpected finding (for example, poor performance indicators or adverse experience or complication of clinical treatment) and is developed because of a desire for change. The aims of the observed practice having been determined, the setting of standards seems much simpler. The pattern described links the audit and learning cycles (fig 3) without appreciably changing either. It might be argued that the learning cycle is much more an individual phenomenon and the operational aspects are related

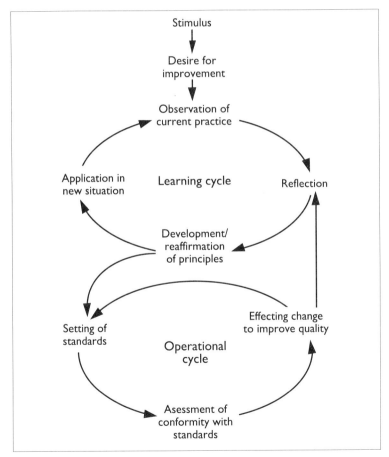

FIG 3—Integration of learning and audit cycles

more to the activities of a clinical team. However, this will probably vary according to the clinical problem under review. Either cycle may stimulate ideas for research and should enhance, not restrict, novel thinking or practice.

Doctor-patient relationships

Audit should not deal solely with outcome measures or use of resources but also with the access to and process of clinical care, which greatly concern the doctor-patient relationship and communication skills. These topics have been given more attention in the recent past by general practitioners and by the practice of reviewing video recordings of a doctor's approach to a patient and his or her presenting history. The nature of such interviews has been shown to alter objective measurements of the quality of care of chronic disease. In diabetic patients when outpatient visits were characterised by meaningful questioning and interruption by the patient the glycated haemoglobin concentration and blood pressure were noted to be lower.[12] Such results may lead to consideration of the doctor-patient relationship as a topic for audit and not merely concerned with consumer satisfaction. The techniques entailed, however, are those of the social scientist, and not many doctors are happy with the approaches of critical incident technique, Delphi techniques, and ethnography; audit may broaden our knowledge of social sciences.

Conclusions

Within the complex relations of medical audit with education some key points emerge:

● Audit is essentially an educational rather than a managerial tool but requires an impetus for learning, a desire for improvement, or quest for excellence
● Learning based on experience and reflection on experience is more effective than study of theory
● Doctors will need to use team leadership skills to create those improvements in quality care that are indicated by audit findings
● District medical education committees will need to learn to exploit the learning opportunities arising from audit
● Audit will require the use of social science skills as well as those currently used.

Finally, medical audit alone poses an exciting challenge for education and will lead to improvements in the quality of clinical care.

1 Secretaries of State for Health, Wales, Northern Ireland, and Scotland. *Medical audit. Working paper 6*. London: HMSO, 1989.
2 Royal College of Physicians. *Medical audit—a first report: what, why and how?* London: RCP, 1989.
3 Royal College of Surgeons. *Guidelines to clinical audit in surgical practice*. London: RCS, 1989.
4 Alment EAJ. *Competence to practise: a report of a committee of inquiry for the medical profession in the United Kingdom*. London: Committee of Inquiry into Competence to Practise, 1976.
5 Adair J. *Action centred leadership*. Aldershot: Gower, 1979.
6 Council for Postgraduate Medical Education in England and Wales. A proposal for a district medical education structure. London: CPME, 1987.
7 Harden R. The curriculum for the year 2000. *Medical Education* 1989;**23**:301–4.
8 Brown G, Atkins M. *Effective teaching in health education*. London: Methuen, 1989.
9 Schon DA. *The reflective practitioner: how professionals think in action*. New York: Basic Books, 1983.
10 Kolb DA. *Experiential learning: experiences as a source of learning and development*. Englewood Cliffs, New Jersey: Prentice Hall, 1984.
11 Coles C. Making audit truly educational. *Postgrad Med J* 1990;**66**(suppl 3):S32–6.
12 Kaplan SH, Greenfield S, Ware JE. Impact of the doctor patient relationship on the outcomes of chronic disease. In: Steward M, Roter D, eds. *Communicating with medical patients*. London: Sage, 1989:228–45.

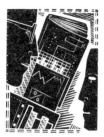

A form to help learn and teach about assessing medical audit papers

RAJ S BHOPAL,
RICHARD THOMSON

The current prominence of medical audit has stimulated publication of papers on the subject and has created a need for a structured and critical approach for reading them. Several guides to the skills required for focused and critical reading of medical publications are available (see, for example, further reading listed in the paper by Fowkes and Fulton[1]); and the analysis of research papers has been particularly well addressed.[1-3] Sackett and colleagues have provided guidance on the analysis of papers on quality of care and other issues relevant to medical audit.[3] However, though these general guidelines are necessary for critical reading of published work on medical audit, we have found them insufficient.

What do we do?
Do we do what we think we do?
What should we do?
Are we doing what we should be doing?
How can we improve what we do?
Have we improved?

BOX 1—Key questions in medical audit

Medical audit is a process for the critical analysis of medical practice, and its essential aim is to improve the quality of routine

178

medical care provided for patients. The essence of medical audit has been summarised by many; it is encapsulated in the questions in box 1 and the audit cycle (see box 2). Unlike research, it is not essential that medical audit extends the knowledge base of medicine. In fact, medical audit is heavily dependent on published data and consensus views. Unlike original research, audit is mainly concerned with assessing and changing routine medical practice and improving standards. Therefore, the emphasis of a critique of published medical audit needs to differ from that of research.

In many instances medical audit is primarily of local value, but sometimes the methods or the findings may be generalisable. If so, the audit deserves dissemination, potentially through publication. The ideal features of a medical audit project suitable for publication, in our view, include the following:

- The topic for study should concern routine medical practice or an aspect of health care which impinges on medical practice
- Standards of practice should preferably be made explicit or, if implicit, should be clearly discernible
- Measurements must be valid, suitable for routine medical practice, and relevant to the standards set
- Assessment of whether clinical standards have been met should be made and, if not, change instituted
- Effects of the change should be evaluated
- Reappraisal of medical practice should occur until the quality of care rises to or exceeds the standards agreed or agreement is reached on a revision of standards, thus creating an audit spiral.

We prepared a form, based on these perspectives, to help read and assess medical audit papers for a regional workshop on audit. We asked each clinician at the workshop to do the following: "List the main features, in your opinion, of a publication on an audit project. In particular consider those features which might induce change in your own practice, or entice you to begin a similar audit of your own practice." We also asked clinicians to comment on the assessment form and to give their opinion on the importance of the individual questions. We subsequently modified the form on the basis of their views on the important attributes of a medical audit paper (table) and from their collated comments on the value of the questions included in the form. The form was subsequently used in the analysis of five papers[4-8] and subsequent discussion of two

		Yes	No	Don't Know/ Not Sure
A Background issues				
1	Is this audit relevant to the quality of patient care?	☐	☐	☐
2	Is the indication for undertaking the audit made explicit?	☐	☐	☐
3	(a) Does the audit investigate routine practice?	☐	☐	☐
	If not:			
	(b) Does the audit concern a non-standard, new or experimental procedure?	☐	☐	☐
4	Does the audit concern a clinical issue characterised by:			
	(a) High volume workload?	☐	☐	☐
	(b) High cost?	☐	☐	☐
	(c) Local or wider concern?	☐	☐	☐
	(d) High variability in practice?	☐	☐	☐
5	(a) Is there consensus or partial consensus on the ideal mode of practice?	☐	☐	☐
	If not:			
	(b) Is it realistic, at the present time, to attempt to develop a consensus on this issue?	☐	☐	☐
6	Is the audit of:			
	(a) Structure of care?	☐	☐	☐
	(b) Process of care?	☐	☐	☐
	(c) Outcome of care?	☐	☐	☐
B Methodological issues				
1	Which, if any, of the following audit designs/approaches is used:			
	(a) Case note review	☐	☐	☐
	(b) Critical incident discussion	☐	☐	☐
	(c) Critical incident monitoring	☐	☐	☐
	(d) Routine data monitoring	☐	☐	☐
	(e) Criterion based topic audit	☐	☐	☐
	(f) Other	☐	☐	☐
	If so, briefly describe:			
2	(a) Are the standards made explicit?	☐	☐	☐
	If not:			
	(b) Are the standards implicit?	☐	☐	☐
3	Is the process of standard setting described?	☐	☐	☐
4	(a) Were standards taken from external sources (for example, medical reports)?	☐	☐	☐
	(b) Were standards adapted from external sources?	☐	☐	☐
	(c) Were standards developed by the authors?	☐	☐	☐
5	Was the audit based on aggregated data?	☐	☐	☐
6	Is the data collection method one that can be used by most clinicians?	☐	☐	☐
7	Are the methods described well enough for you to repeat the audit?	☐	☐	☐
8	(a) Are the results compared explicitly with standards?	☐	☐	☐
	If not:			
	(b) Are the results compared implicitly with standards?	☐	☐	☐

C Implications for clinical practice

1. Do the authors indicate whether practice needs to be altered? ☐ ☐ ☐
2. Are you convinced by their arguments? ☐ ☐ ☐
3. Are appropriate and realistic changes suggested? ☐ ☐ ☐
4. Are the resource implications of the changes discussed? ☐ ☐ ☐
5. Were the suggested changes implemented? ☐ ☐ ☐
6. Were the changes described well enough for them to be implemented in your hospital/setting? ☐ ☐ ☐
7. Was the impact of change evaluated? ☐ ☐ ☐
8. (a) Did the change lead to the anticipated benefit? ☐ ☐ ☐
   If not:
   (b) Were the reasons discussed? ☐ ☐ ☐
9. (a) Were the benefits sustained? ☐ ☐ ☐
   If not:
   (b) Were the reasons discussed? ☐ ☐ ☐
10. Were the standards revised as a result of the audit? ☐ ☐ ☐
11. Were areas requiring educational input identified? ☐ ☐ ☐
12. Were opportunities for future audit projects identified? ☐ ☐ ☐
13. Were opportunities for research identified? ☐ ☐ ☐

Consider the audit cycle below and indicate how far this report has progressed around the cycle

Measure baseline

Set standards

Review standards

Measure practice

Evaluate change

Compare against standards

Implement change

Identify opportunity for improvement

Suggest change

If you have any further general comments about the audit report not covered by the above questions please make them below:

Views on important attributes of medical audit papers among 25 clinicians attending regional workshop on audit

Category and description of attributes		No of mentions
Topic		32
Routine, relevant, practical	14	
High volume, may save time and money, high cost	11	
Practice needs change	5	
Local concern or interest	2	
Aims		11
Clear objectives	5	
Focused audit on simple question	6	
Standards		11
Standards, criteria, guidelines made clear	8	
Process for setting standards clear or realistic	3	
Measurements		12
Methods easy, repeatable, clear, sound	12	
Interpretation		11
All factors leading to change considered	8	
Statistical analysis included	3	
Benefits and outcomes		16
Benefits shown in terms of health—for example, mortality	9	
Benefits (unspecified)	2	
Outcomes measured	5	
Implementation		16
Change easy or within existing resources	6	
Change made or audit cycle completed	7	
Resource implication of audit and its implementation discussed	2	
Change sustainable	1	
Others		5
Educational value	1	
Acceptable to colleagues	1	
Cross specialty work	1	
Patient satisfaction considered	2	

papers[7 8] on audit with two groups of lead clinicians (local medical audit committee chairman and specialty audit lead clinicians) and two groups of clinicians with an emerging interest in audit.

Content and purpose of assessment form

The form is in four parts: background issues, methodological issues, implications for medical practice, and a diagram of the audit cycle on which the reader marks the characteristics of the paper.

The completion of the form and subsequent discussion of it in an open forum of clinicians were intended to:

● Develop and refine a structured approach that could be applied to any published paper on medical audit (and, potentially, to unpublished audit projects and protocols)

● Provoke consideration, from first principles, of what to expect an audit paper to contain and hence to reinforce clinicians' understanding of the nature and purpose of audit

● Provide an opportunity of analysing several recent illustrative publications

● Reinforce the main principles of medical audit and illustrate that some principles are not fixed but evolving, through the discussion of the varying responses given by clinicians

● Engender debate on issues such as standards, criteria, and guidelines by discussing a paper's content and highlighting areas of uncertainty.

The form helped to achieve these objectives, as evidenced by feedback from the clinicians: 38 of 74 participants in the workshops subsequently completed an evaluation questionnaire (some are still expected), 34 of whom stated that they felt better able to assess and criticise audit reports; all but one clinician reported that the session in which the form had been used was valuable.

Discussion

The rapid pace of medical progress requires doctors to read original research reports and not to rely only on textbooks. As many writers have emphasised, reading original reports is best performed in a critical and structured approach. In this way, as Sackett and colleagues clearly showed,[3] doctors may avoid being misled by spurious findings and use their reading time more effectively. Sackett and colleagues provided short accounts of how to read papers on a range of issues, including a few questions on the quality of care. We are unaware, however, of a comprehensive, structured approach to reading which concerns the specific attributes of medical audit papers.

Presently, many doctors need to learn quickly the principles and techniques of medical audit. Their need for continuing education in medical audit will be met not only by short courses and practical experience but also by reading the emerging publications on medical audit. Medical audit projects, unlike general research, will often exhort (explicitly or implicitly) change in medical practice.

In these circumstances doctors need to consider carefully the nature, validity, generalisability, and applicability of the work. Combined with previously published guidelines for critical appraisal of research, our form provides an approach for doctors to do this. In the process of systematically analysing papers doctors can consolidate their knowledge on the nature of medical audit. We emphasise that our form is part of a reading "toolkit" and cannot alone lead to a valid appraisal of the scientific validity of the paper (question C2 for example, requires general appraisal skills). In our experience the form is a useful teaching aid and helps to generate discussion on the core elements of a published medical audit paper. The form may also be useful for reviewing manuscripts and outlines of medical audit projects and for doctors designing audit projects, but as yet we have no practical experience of these uses.

Medical audit papers are not unique in addressing issues relating to the quality of medical care, and, combined with other reading aids, parts of our form—for example, section C—may be useful to clinicians in assessing other types of publication.

Our form was prepared on the basis of first principles and subsequently modified. We believe that it is reasonably comprehensive and, on the basis of the data in the table, that it focuses on the issues within medical audit papers which clinicians deem to be important. The clinicians at the workshops reported that audit publications, particularly those which might influence their own practice, should include a focus on routine, high volume medical care, be concerned with simple questions, use straightforward methods, and place emphasis on the implementation of change. They did not emphasise educational value or patient satisfaction as important attributes of published audit. The last two observations surprised us and may merit further study and reflection.

In conclusion, papers on medical audit need to be read particularly carefully by doctors who may be influenced to change their medical practice. They should utilise techniques for critical appraisal and a structured approach. Our form is an adjunct to established methods for learning and teaching about medical audit.

1 Fowkes FGR, Fulton PM. Critical appraisal of published research: introductory guidelines. *BMJ* 1991;**302**:1136–40.
2 Easterbrook P. "Critical appraisal" or how to interpret journal articles. *BMJ* 1990; **302**:392–3.
3 Sackett DL, Haynes RB, Tugwell P. *Clinical epidemiology. A basic science for clinical medicine*. Boston: Little, Brown, 1985.

4 Hancock BD. Audit of major colorectal and biliary surgery to reduce rates of wound infection. *BMJ* 1990;**301**:911–2.
5 Rutherford AD. Blood usage and laminectomy. *J R Coll Surg Edinb* 1987;**32**:72–3.
6 Neville RG. Notifying general practitioners about deaths in hospital: an audit. *J R Coll Gen Pract* 1987;**37**:496–7.
7 Milne RIG. Assessment of care in children with sickle cell disease: implications for neonatal screening programmes. *BMJ* 1990;**300**:371–4.
8 Fowkes FGR, Hall R, Jones JH, Scanlon MF, Elder GH, Hobbs DR, *et al.* Trial of strategy for reducing the use of laboratory tests. *BMJ* 1986;**292**:883–5.

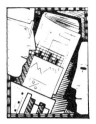

TOWARDS ACHIEVING QUALITY

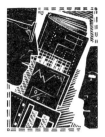

Algorithm based improvement of clinical quality

STEPHEN C SCHOENBAUM,
LAWRENCE K GOTTLIEB

Ambulatory medical practice has traditionally taken place behind closed office doors. In recent years there has been a shift of important clinical decision making from the hospital setting to the physician's office, and ambulatory practices have been organised into managed entities (for example, health maintenance organisations and large group practices). Concomitantly, there has been an increasing interest in managing the practice that occurs behind the closed office door without violating the confidentiality of the physician-patient relationship. Problems relating to widespread variation in practices and practice styles have begun to surface, and the issue is not whether, but how best, to manage the variation. One approach, which is increasingly discussed, is to develop guidelines for practice. Though developing and disseminating guidelines undoubtedly will be increasingly important in managing clinical practices, guidelines are just the initial component of a cyclical process for improving clinical performance.

In this article we illustrate some of the clinical management issues that managers face; provide a general framework for dealing with those problems, which includes developing and implementing practice guidelines; give a specific example of a clinical quality improvement project in our own organisation; and make some general points about the opportunities and difficulties of this approach.

Clinical management issues

Consider the treatment of a common situation such as prescribing oral contraceptives. About 20 different brand names are marketed in the United States, each with various formulations and dosages. One advantage of an organisation of managed care is that it should be able to purchase pharmaceuticals in high volume at a favourable price and pass the savings to its patients. How can the organisation influence the physician to write for a limited number of products? How does it obtain the desired behaviour without interfering with the "best judgment" of the physician?

Consider a different problem. Two patients, who are friends, have the same clinical condition but are treated differently by two physicians who work for the same health care organisation. One patient has a bad outcome. The friends compare notes and discover the difference in the way they were handled and in their outcomes. The one with the bad outcome asks the management of the health care organisation to explain the difference. Though the difference really may not be explainable, the management often states that there are many different "acceptable" ways to handle the same problem. Yet, if care is managed, shouldn't there have been careful consideration of the benefits, risks, and costs of treatment by the physicians in the organisation? Shouldn't those physicians have concluded either that there is an optimal approach or that several approaches are equally acceptable? Should the organisation tolerate unexplained variation in care when it is potentially liable for the poor outcomes?

Process of clinical quality improvement

Such considerations in 1985 led Harvard Community Health Plan, a large health maintenance organisation in the Boston area of Massachusetts, to initiate an activity for developing and implementing clinical standards or guidelines.[1] Although guidelines may be useful for the retrospective assessment of care, we wanted to develop tools and programmes to assist or support clinicians in delivering appropriate care. In this context we consider a guideline to be just one part of a support system for managing clinical care. Our guidelines have usually taken the form of algorithms, as the process of care is often best described by a linked series of "if . . . then" statements. The basic elements of the clinical quality improvement process may be broken down into four distinct phases (box). Once a particular clinical process is selected for quality improvement a team of clinicians and managers is assembled and the focus of the project is clarified. The team then

---

The clinical quality improvement process

Definition and organisation of project
List and prioritise problems
Define project and team

Development of guidelines
Identify relevant individuals and assess their needs
Consider scientific evidence
Consider clinical experience
Consider outcomes and preferences
Develop consensus guidelines

Problem prevention and implementation
Consider potential problems and causes
Develop support systems for prevention
Design measurement system
Implement guideline and systems supports

Measurement and evaluation
Measure performance: process and outcomes
Monitor systems

---

proceeds to analyse the problem, identify the relevant staff involved in the care process, and develop a consensus guideline based on the available scientific evidence and the group's clinical experience. Once the guideline is completed the group must consider potential barriers to the faithful execution of the care plans specified by the guideline and design a strategy to overcome those barriers. Potential problem areas may be related to the knowledge and skills of the clinician, the capabilities of the delivery system, and the overall practice environment. Preventive measures may include publication and distribution of the guideline, focused education programmes, automated and manual decision support systems (including clinical reminder systems), and administrative mechanisms. Once the preventive measures are specified, key quality indicators are identified and a measurement plan is designed. After the new clinical guidelines and systems supports are implemented performance is measured and another round of the quality improvement cycle is initiated as appropriate.

Clinical quality improvement in screening for cervical cancer

Cervical cancer screening by the use of the Papanicolaou smear is a common and important procedure in ambulatory care. When considering the quality of care for female patients who undergo cervical cytological screening attention usually has been directed to the quality of the laboratory reading the smear. The overall process, however, consists of multiple steps, each of which must be carried out properly to assure high quality care. The steps include obtaining specimens at the appropriate intervals from the entire population at risk, obtaining specimens that are most suitable for reading, handling them so that they get to the laboratory promptly in good condition, reading them accurately and expeditiously, notifying the clinician of the results appropriately, notifying the patient, and performing suitable follow up care for women with an abnormal result.

We have tried to assess and, if necessary, modify each step in this process: the department of quality of care measurement at the Harvard Community Health Plan performs surveys of screening practices among our members by reviewing medical records. In 1989, for example, in Harvard Community Health Plan's health centres division, an organisation which delivers care to over 300 000 members at 12 sites, 92% of new female members who had an initial health assessment were recorded to have had a pelvic examination and smear, and 76% of a random sample of women who had been members for at least one year had had a Papanicolaou smear recorded in the previous two years. This practice is supported by an automated reminder system that, for every routine primary care encounter, prints out an age-sex specific listing of recommended screening practices.[2] There is possible room for improvement at this step as we still may be missing women who have not had a visit and may be screening others more often than necessary.

The Harvard Community Health Plan's central cytology laboratory is processing almost 100 000 smears annually. The laboratory is accredited and has a strong quality control programme. Though there has been considerable concern in recent years about the accuracy of readings in many cytology laboratories, our concerns were primarily directed to the processes of acquiring and following up smears. Endocervical elements (endocervical glandular cells and squamous metaplastic cells) were present in only 37–45% of the smears, and we found that there was substantial variation in the techniques by which specimens were being obtained. Though a trial of training in optimal technique improved the rate of endocervical elements present to 70%, a working group of our internists and gynaecologists convened to develop guidelines for cervical cancer screening practices and follow up ultimately recommended use of endocervical brushes to improve the yield of endocervical elements even more and avoid the need for

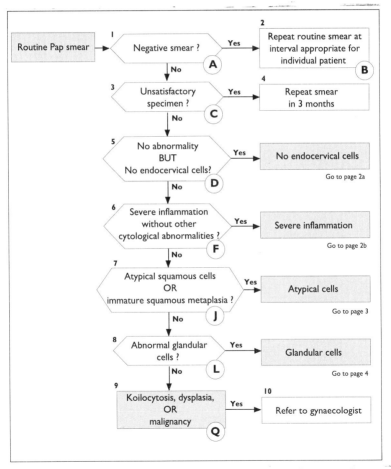

FIG 1—Evaluation and management of abnormal Papanicolaou (Pap) smear by primary care providers (March 1989)

many repeat smears. Implementing this technique by in service education and including the brush in the equipment for pelvic examinations increased the rate of recovery of endocervical elements to 87–89% with an appreciable decrease in variation among clinicians.

The working group developed algorithms for evaluating and managing abnormal smears by primary care providers (fig 1) and by gynaecologists. Figure 1 shows the overall algorithm, and figure 2 shows the portion of the algorithm specifying follow up of patients with abnormal glandular cells.

The practical question is how to help physicians do the follow up steps in the table and do them uniformly. We chose to support the implementation of this algorithm by programming our laboratory system with a set of prompts. Accordingly, when an abnormal cervical smear test result is reported from the laboratory to the physician the report contains a statement of the follow up recommended by the algorithm (a prompt). This process dovetails with a reminder system, which in turn is linked to our COSTAR based

Algorithm summary of evaluation and management of abnormal Papanicolaou (Pap) smear by primary care providers (March 1989)

Papanicolaou result	Recommended follow up
Negative	Repeat routine smear at interval appropriate for individual patient (Box 1, annotations A and B)
Unsatisfactory	Repeat smear in 3 months (Box 3, annotation C)
No abnormality, BUT no endocervical cells	Repeat smear in 3 months or one year depending on results of previous smears (Box 5, annotations D and E)
Severe inflammation without other cytological abnormalities	Consider treatment for infectious agents or atrophic changes as indicated (Box 6, annotations F–I)
Atypical squamous cells OR immature squamous metaplasia	Treat any identified infections or atrophic changes. Repeat smear every 3 months, twice. Refer to gynaecologist if either repeat smear is abnormal (Box 7, annotations J and K)
Endometrial cells	If patient is postmenopausal refer to gynaecologist, if premenopausal repeat smear at mid-cycle and refer if endometrial cells persist (Boxes 8 and 29, annotations M–O)
Atypical endocervical cells	Evaluate and treat for possible infectious aetiologies. Repeat smear in 3 months. Refer to gynaecologist if atypical endocervical cells persist (Boxes 8 and 34, annotation P)
Koilocytosis, dysplasia, or malignancy	Refer to gynaecologist (Box 9, annotation Q)

automated medical record system.[2] The record system periodically searches the records of patients with abnormal smear test results to determine if the first follow up step has occurred in the appropriate time interval. If not the physician is notified. Reminders such as these circumvent problems which arise because the original laboratory result was lost or ignored by the clinician or patient. Data from our department of quality of care measurement indicate that only two thirds of patients with abnormalities on smear testing have had an appropriate follow up recorded within the first three months; by six months, however, 99% have had an appropriate follow up. Given the volume of activity, the remaining 1% represents almost 50 patients a year with an abnormal smear who have not had appropriate follow up. Accordingly, we instituted a manual reminder system for the residual 1% and now know that we have notified or treated all patients with abnormal smear test results.

General comments

The example of cervical cancer screening gives some notion of the complexity of managing medical care, even for ostensibly simple and common issues. Is it worth the effort to go through the process of developing and implementing algorithm based or guideline based approaches to care? In general, we believe that it is, for several reasons.

Specifying the overall process of care allows logical assessment and improvement of its components. It draws attention to opportunities to improve quality that tend otherwise to be overlooked— that is, improving screening and follow up performance, not just focusing on technical aspects of preparing and reading smears in the laboratory.

The development of algorithms or guidelines by clinicians has educational importance within health care systems. Much knowledge of ambulatory practice has not been shared. When the sharing occurs better ideas arise. Additionally, group work on developing or modifying a guideline leads to its local ratification, an important first step in its implementation.

Developing the algorithm itself does not necessarily ensure improved performance. Nevertheless, the nature of the support systems and measures necessary to improve and monitor performance become apparent. Systems and technologies—for example, use of endocervical brushes—may improve care directly. Measurement not only indicates the success of the intervention but may also be an intervention itself. It provides important feedback to physicians, and feedback is itself a way of improving performance.

Specification of process decreases variation. It leads to standardisation of practices and techniques which can decrease error, waste, rework, and unit cost. When all parties know what to expect it is easier to facilitate the correct procedure and to monitor for error. In our example of cervical cytology screening, standardisation of the use of endocervical brushes permitted the brushes to be included routinely in the equipment for the pelvic examination, which led to greater recovery of endocervical elements and to fewer return visits to collect a better sample. By having achieved agreement on a standard technique we can now develop standardised educational materials to explain to patients the exact nature of the procedure they can expect to undergo; and if a new process

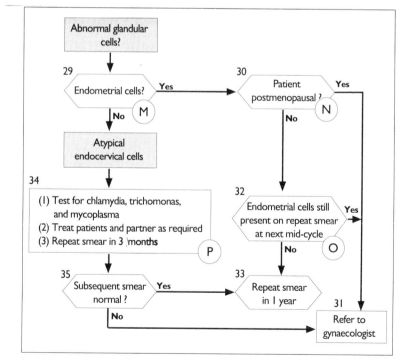

FIG 2—Management for abnormal glandular cells

improvement is proposed we will be able to compare it with a known standard technique rather than unknown and varying techniques.

On the other hand, the development of guidelines and systems to support them is time consuming, and the expenditures of creating the guidelines and systems are apparent before the savings. It may be necessary to implement automated information systems to facilitate many desirable clinical process improvements, and few models for these exist. In addition, as it is usual to find that performance of recommended clinical processes is less than 100%[3] the result of improvements in clinical process may be to offset savings in unit costs of services with increased units of service.

Nevertheless, we have reached a critical juncture in health care and now realise that quality of care is not just a function of using more complex technologies. Evaluating and improving the processes of care is not simple, nor is it a task which in the past was highly rewarded. Now that we have opened ourselves to examination and can see the opportunities for process improvement, we will probably adopt the tools for improvement including development of guidelines or process specification, support systems for implementing improved processes, ongoing measurement of how we are doing, and formal reassessments.

1 Gottlieb LK, Margolis CZ, Schoenbaum SC. Clinical practice guidelines at an HMO: development and implementation in a quality improvement model. *Quality Review Bulletin* 1990;**16**:80–6.
2 Schoenbaum SC. Implementation of preventive services in an HMO practice. *J General Intern Med* 1990;**5**:S123–7.
3 Schoenbaum SC. When is the quality of care good enough? *Am J Public Health* 1990; **80**:403–4.

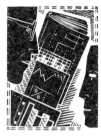

Variations in hospital admissions and the appropriateness of care: American preoccupations?

JOHN P BUNKER

It is not just the explosion in costs that has catalysed preoccupation with the cost effectiveness of medical care in the United States. There is an equally important and growing recognition of the uncertain effectiveness of much of medical care itself, which has emerged directly from the now widely confirmed large and unexplained variations in rates of hospital admissions observed across local, regional, and national populations. Recognition that different segments of the population may receive appreciably different rates of a particular treatment is not new. Glover reported to the Royal College of Physicians in 1938 that rates of tonsillectomy varied as much as 20-fold among school districts in England and Wales.[1] Threefold and fourfold differences in rates for other surgical procedures were observed in Liverpool, New England, and Uppsala by Pearson et al in 1968[2] and among 11 health planning regions in Kansas by Lewis in 1969.[3]

Magnitude of variation

I first became aware that there was a large public health problem a year later, when national data on operation rates in the United States became available and I could compare them with those published by the British Hospital In-Patient Enquiry.[4] People in the United States at that time were twice as likely to undergo surgery as were those in Britain. Whether those in the United States were receiving too much surgery or those in Britain too little was indeterminable. People in the United States had not gained the benefit of living longer; indeed, life expectancy in Great Britain was slightly greater in 1970. Perhaps they were gaining an improvement in the quality of life, a goal to which much of medical and surgical care is devoted, but there were no data to determine this. Life expectancy in the United States is now slightly greater than in Britain, probably owing more to differences in smoking and other lifestyle factors than to medical care. It is still not possible to say whether the quality of life of the average person in the United States is better than that of one in Britain. The magnitude of the problem became painfully apparent in 1973 with the publication by Wennberg and Gittelsohn of large variations in rates of operation among thirteen "small areas," roughly equivalent to counties, in Vermont.[5] Vermont is a rural state with a largely homogeneous population and no discernible differences in morbidity to account for possible differences in medical need. Variations of equal magnitude in rates of operation were subsequently widely confirmed in other states and in other countries, including Great Britain.[6] Variations in hospital admissions for medical diagnoses are even greater in the United States; on the basis of widely reported large variations in general practitioner referrals for consultant care,[7] I judge that they are equally large in Britain. Coulter *et al* have now confirmed large variations in general medical admissions.[7a]

Large variations in hospital admissions might be considered to have very different meanings in the United States and Great Britain. Variations in the United States might be reasonably assumed to include a good deal of overtreatment, and those in Britain, equally large but occurring at considerably lower absolute levels, to represent a good deal of undertreatment. Though these may be valid judgments, the fact that such variations occur in each country is strong evidence that the quality of medical care given by doctors in both is equally variable and uncertain. In the United States a large effort has been made to find the cause of the observed variations in medical practice. Only a small part of the variation has been attributed to variations in the prevalence of disease or to chance statistical variation. Rates of operation have been shown to vary directly with the number of surgeons and rates of admission with the number of beds available, but these explain only part of the effect. More important is the question of how medical decisions to treat similar conditions may vary so greatly among doctors. It is now widely acknowledged that this must mean that the scientific basis of the practice of medicine is inadequate; that the outcomes of treatment are, as a consequence, uncertain; and that, as a further result, doctors disagree among themselves in choosing treatment.[8] There is also a growing body of evidence that doctors may not use existing scientific knowledge to full advantage.

Judging appropriateness of indications for procedures

The need for better data on the outcome of diagnostic and therapeutic technologies has been recognised for many years, but a national effort to respond to this need has only recently been implemented in the United States and given appropriate funds. A new agency for health care policy and research, with a budget for the current fiscal year of $100m, was created by the United States Congress in December 1989. The agency is charged with the responsibility "to enhance the quality, appropriateness, and effectiveness of health care services . . . through the establishment of a broad base of scientific research and through the promotion of improvements in clinical practice and in the organization, financing, and delivery of health care services." Resolution of the uncertainty underlying variations in rates of hospital care was the major rationale for creating the agency.

The need to use existing data more effectively is also widely acknowledged: the effectiveness of medical care in general falls far short of the best of which medical care is capable. Considerable effort has been made, primarily in the United States, to lessen the gap between care as practised on average and care provided under optimal conditions. Quality assurance programmes, including medical audit, represent one such effort. Consensus conferences, implemented by the National Institutes of Health in 1977, represent another. These conferences convene "a carefully selected panel of persons thought to be without vested interest, to listen to the evidence presented . . . and to prepare a report on the topic under consideration, including recommendations."[9] Panels of experts are now being used, in a somewhat similar manner as in the consensus conferences, to judge the "appropriateness" of the indications for various medical and surgical procedures,[10] the results of which are being used, in turn, as a basis for granting or withholding payment for care. The potential for similar use of data on appropriateness of care in negotiations of NHS contracts is currently under review at the King's Fund Centre (D W Costain, personal communication).

Perhaps the most interesting response to the phenomenon of variation and to the underlying implied uncertainty has been the substantial amount of research by health policy analysts of the transfer of scientific data to clinical practice and of how medical decisions are made, together with a ground swell of self examination by the medical profession as a whole. The Institute of Medicine in Washington last year held two conferences on improving the translation of research findings into clinical practice, clearly the weakest link in the process of medical innovation. Adoption of new medical technology seems to have as much to do with medical leadership and precedent in a given place as with its demonstrated efficacy. Standards of practice for old procedures, as well as for new, set by "opinion leaders" of a medical community are thought to explain the phenomenon of variation. That each medical community may have quite different clinical policies or standards is attributed to the uncertainty surrounding much of medical practice. Variations in care should diminish as local standards are replaced by national standards. Consensus conferences represent an important step in the effort to establish such national standards but are limited by the adequacy of the scientific base they attempt to synthesise and by the bias of the "experts" convened. Research on outcomes, or the "evaluative clinical sciences" as they are starting to be called in the United States, will continue to be the central necessary ingredient in the effort to improve clinical practice.

Common problems and solutions

The United States and Britain have a common medical goal based on a common problem, and despite the appreciable differences in how medical care is organised and paid for the solution is also a common one. The goal is improvement in the care of patients within existing economic constraints. The solution is a better scientific base readily accessible to clinicians in their practice of medicine.[11]

Quality assurance programmes, medical audit, and, now, assessment of the appropriateness of care represent the major current efforts to improve care by attempting to eliminate care of poor quality. A good beginning, perhaps; a necessary first step, probably; but in the process of rooting out the "bad apples" we have largely neglected the need to measure and encourage good medical care.[12] It is important to bear in mind that in identifying poor quality care we cannot assume that the remainder is good; that identifying and minimising adverse drug reactions does not assure that when such reaction does not occur the drug is achieving the purpose for which it was prescribed; and that when we have eliminated those diagnostic and therapeutic procedures that are judged to be clearly inappropriate we still do not know how many of the residual "appropriate" and "equivocal" procedures are achieving their intended results.

"Not bad" medicine does not equal good medicine, and we have only begun to face the enormous task of measuring at a population level the positive impact of medical care, encompassing how much good medicine does overall and how much good it does procedure by procedure and condition by condition. This is the task to which the new agency in Washington is committed and for which Congress has appropriated what may seem like a large sum of money, but which will, in all likelihood, cost much more. And even this is only half the job, for to make the results of research on outcomes readily available to practising clinicians—a goal implicit in the British government's commitment to a nationwide information system as part of *Working for Patients*[13]—it will be necessary to invest equally large, and as yet unestimated, sums of money.

1 Glover JA. The incidence of tonsillectomy in school children. *Proc R Soc Med* 1938;**31**:1219–36.

2 Pearson RJC, Smedby B, Berfenstam R, Logan RFL, Burgess AM, Peterson OL. Hospital caseloads in Liverpool, New England and Uppsala: an international comparison. *Lancet* 1968;ii:559–66.

3 Lewis CE. Variations in the incidence of surgery. *N Engl J Med* 1969;**281**:880–4.

4 Bunker JP. Surgical manpower: a comparison of operations and surgeons in the United States and in England and Wales. *N Engl J Med* 1970;**282**:135–44.

5 Wennberg JE, Gittelsohn A. Small area variations in health care delivery: a population-based health information system can guide planning and regulatory decision-making. *Science* 1973;**182**:1102–8.

6 McPherson K, Wennberg JE, Hovind OB, Clifford P. Small-area variations in the use of common surgical procedures: an international comparison of New England, England and Norway. *N Engl J Med* 1982;**307**:1310–4.

7 Dowie R. *General practitioners and consultants: a study of outpatient referrals.* London: King Edward's Hospital Fund for London, 1983.

7a Coulter A, Seagrott A, McPherson K. Relation between general practices' outpatient referral rates and rates of elective admission to hospital. *Br Med J* 1990;**301**:273–7.

8 Bunker JP. When doctors disagree. *New York Review of Books* 1985;April 25:7.
9 Perry S. The NIH consensus development program: a decade later. *N Engl J Med* 1987;**317**:485–8.
10 Park RE, Fink A, Brook RH, *et al.* Physician ratings of appropriate indications for six medical and surgical procedures. *Am J Publ Health* 1986;**76**:766–72.
11 McPherson K, Bunker JP. Health information as a guide to the organization and delivery of services. In: Holland WW, Knox G, Detels R, eds. *Oxford textbook of public health*. Oxford: Oxford University Press (in press).
12 Berwick DM. Continuous improvement as an ideal in health care. *N Engl J Med* 1989;**320**:53–6.
13 Secretaries of State for Health, Wales, Northern Ireland, and Scotland. *Working for patients*. London: HMSO, 1989. (Cm 555.)

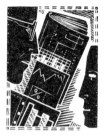

Arcadia revisited: quality assurance in hospitals in The Netherlands

EVERT REERINK

Of all the attributes of medical care the assurance of its quality is the least known. At best it is respected, but it is never loved and never popular. Scientific progress, medical research, eradication of disease, and alleviation of grief and sorrow continue to be the pinnacles of medical care. Accountability, openness, and empathy do not score highly. Yet these are equally traditional values of the medical profession that must be taught, disseminated, and, often, defended.

Medicine as it is practised is as much engrained in a country's culture and tradition as are, say, literature and the arts. If the intellectual and political climates are favourable to, or at least tolerant of, the development of arts and sciences, medical care will profit—and this holds true for quality assurance. The keys to the proper development of modern quality assurance are tolerance, common consent, and confidence. Conflict, mistrust, and competition are definitely counterproductive. Each country has the quality assurance system that befits its health care system.

Dutch health care system

In The Netherlands it seemed appropriate to hold physicians responsible for their professional work, and on this basis they claimed responsibility for the quality of their care, the ultimate consequence of which is to assess quality and, if necessary, improve it. Assessing and improving quality is relatively recent. In the 1960s and early 1970s few professionals bothered. Around 1975, however, hospital doctors, united in their national specialists organisation, Landelijke Specialisten Vereniging, and perhaps triggered by the developments in the United States, where state organisations (Professional Standards Review Organizations) had been established to look into the quality of medical care in hospitals, and by the realisation that the current methods of quality care assurance were hopelessly outdated, renewed the tenet that physicians must be responsible for their quality of work. The Landelijke Specialisten Vereniging also took the next step: though professing their responsibility, specialists also acknowledged their ignorance of how to conduct modern quality assurance. Help and support were necessary.[1] The government fell in with the idea for this initiative, leaving professional quality assurance to the health professions and supporting the creation of CBO, an organisation to help clinicians in their self imposed task of quality assurance. The government completed the so called tripod of quality assurance by declaring openly its non-interference in quality assurance in the health care sector and instead professed its commitment to the cause. It and subsequent governments were set on a course of diminished interference in health care, and the new proposal fell on fertile ground. However, all parties thought that something should be done about the perceived unattained benefit in medical care.

Present problems in health care

At that time the Dutch health care system, which had previously been in good shape, started to show several shortcomings. This was not unique: the health care system in The Netherlands had (and has) similar problems to those of health care systems in other developed countries. There is considerable similarity between the health care problems in The Netherlands and Britain: increasing health care costs, an uncontrollable influx of expensive and often potentially dangerous technology, an increasing number of industrial disputes involving salaried nurses and physicians working on a fee for service basis, often vociferous public indignation, increasing numbers of patient claims, and attacks on health care in the press. In medicine itself problems were perceived, such as a lack of effectiveness, courtesy, and information to patients; uninformative medical records; and unsatisfactory communication between professionals. It is also clear that the solutions to these problems are similar in both countries: to re-establish working relations between professionals and both the government and hospital management, increase collaboration between professions, introduce patients as equal partners in matters pertaining to their health and disease, stem the flood of mishaps, and generally improve the quality of care delivery. Still the question remains of how to go about this.

Quality assurance

In most of the issues above quality of care (or its lack) was the core of the problem and had to be addressed squarely. Although a support organisation had been created, it remained primarily the task of the professionals to improve their quality of work. Thus in the hospitals quality assurance committees were set up and programmes were designed to address the most obvious and prevalent problems with quality. By their nature these problems differed from hospital to hospital: from more than 1400 priority problems selected in 46 hospitals between 1977 and 1990 about a third were typically problems of effectiveness—doctors could achieve better outcomes and increase the benefit for their patients; a third could be called problems of efficiency—doctors could better make use of the existing resources; and the remaining third was a conglomerate of patient related problems and organisational and interpersonal problems (conflicts) that needed to be solved among professionals. The same divisions pertain to nursing and physiotherapy, which are two recent additions to hospital quality assurance targets.

One basic method for assuring quality

In The Netherlands the term health care quality assurance is preferred to terms indicating its separate elements, such as medical audit or nursing audit, reflecting willingness to break down interprofessional barriers and recognise health care as a joint venture in which many professionals participate and collaborate.

To make things clear to busy clinicians the method of quality assurance was introduced in the simplest of terms, and clinicians were presented with one basic methodological framework (figure). This problem solving method looks just like medical practice in its assessment and improvement constituents. With this framework it is easy to determine what the various tasks are, where a division of

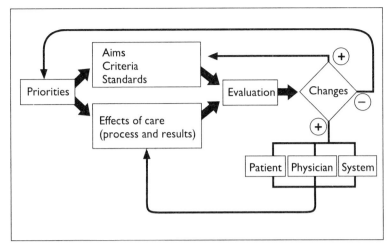

Steps in quality assurance process

tasks is in order, and where the emphasis should be. It has been applied in all health care sectors where quality of care is a concern: since 1974 in a growing number of acute care hospitals; in general practice (since 1980 through a separate support organisation); in nursing (since 1984), physiotherapy (since 1988), and other para-medical services; and in future in mental health (from 1991) and occupational health. Nevertheless, the main focus up to now has been on hospital care.

Practice of quality assurance

In acute care hospitals and most university hospitals many quality assurance activities have been effected since the declaration of the Landelijke Specialisten Vereniging and the inception of CBO. Local quality assurance committees, which are often multi-disciplinary, set their own programme to deal with their own problems of quality.[2] In a few hospitals quality assurance professionals, mostly physicians, have joined the committees to alleviate their tasks. The table shows a sample of study topics.

In keeping with the underlying thought of the quality assurance programme, consultant doctors are the mainstay of the job, being engaged in either running the programme (which generally takes one 90 minute planning and coordination meeting every three

---

Sample problems for quality assurance activity in a general hospital

Preoperative assessment in ASA-I* patients
Prevention of decubitus (bed sores)
Accuracy of execution of dietary prescriptions
Elimination of side effects after gentamicin treatment
Need for skull radiographs after skull trauma
Deficient medical record keeping
Appropriateness of intravenous alimentation
Appropriateness of do not resuscitate policies
Improved triage in the emergency department

*ASA-I = American Society of Anesthesiologists category I (otherwise healthy patients operated on for a minor ailment)

---

professionals. It is also clear that the solutions to these problems are similar in both countries: to re-establish working relations between professionals and both the government and hospital management, increase collaboration between professions, introduce patients as equal partners in matters pertaining to their health and disease, stem the flood of mishaps, and generally improve the quality of care delivery. Still the question remains of how to go about this.

Changes in practice may be observed, although this seems to take time. Studies in which, for example, the proper completion of the medical record has been investigated show that it may take many months before an appreciable change is detected. The need for behavioural change is noted much more commonly than the need for more education.[3] In addition, it must be noted that the medical staff in a hospital, the body which in this quality assurance system is the final arbiter in medical quality issues, is a fairly recently established institution: in some hospitals the medical staff is not yet fully equipped to take the necessary educational and corrective measures expected of it. However, physicians are now more knowledgeable about quality assurance and appreciate that it is not the threatening activity which they had hitherto resisted. Quality assurance in nursing has been even more successful in implementing change, and the same holds true for other disciplines such as physiotherapy.

Towards a national quality assurance policy

The apparent success of quality assurance in hospitals has

encouraged similar activities in other sectors within and outside hospitals, such as dentistry and pharmacy. A national policy was set in 1989 and renewed in 1990 in which health professionals, institutions, financiers, and the government participated. This led to the decision by the Ministry of Health not to introduce prescriptive legislation that might interfere with professional quality assurance matters. Instead it opts for supportive legislation that stimulates quality assurance in all branches of health care.

Resource centre for quality assurance

The existence of CBO, the Utrecht based independent resource centre for quality assurance in hospitals, has triggered discussions on similar institutions in other countries. Invariably attempts were made to copy the centre but were followed by the admission that a resource centre is but one element in the tripod on which modern quality assurance is based, and that its foundation and functioning are highly dependent on suitable staff and stable funding. Yet in some European countries analogous organisations have been built up: in Belgium (Louvain), Germany (Kiel and Munich), Italy (Udine), France (Paris), and Spain (Barcelona and Madrid), often with the active support from The Netherlands. Even countries such as Australia, Malaysia, Canada, and the United States with their tradition of compulsory quality assurance have adopted the philosophy of assisting health care providers in setting up and maintaining voluntary quality assurance activities in hospitals. A recent project of the World Bank aimed at instituting quality assurance in the general hospitals of Bangladesh will start with creating a resource centre in Dhaka, to support clinicians and nurses in executing their new task successfully.

The future

The introduction of quality assurance in any sector of health care should never be a single event, a solo action by an interested party; many more elements must be taken into account, acted on, and attuned to the common goal of improving the quality of health care delivery. Pertinent legislation; a positive attitude of health professionals, hospital management, and politicians; dealing with resistance to change; educating health care professionals and patients; and providing funds are the main elements of a whole fabric, of which the introduction and maintenance of quality assurance is only one part.[4] Thus a resource centre, which can deal with all these issues simultaneously through expertise and networking, is the more necessary. Countries that worry about the quality of their hospital services might start with creating such an independent centre and enjoy the benefits it brings.

There is unanimity in The Netherlands about the course of quality assurance for the coming years. But all parties acknowledge the difficulties entailed in upholding the fabric as it has been developed in the past 10 years. The Arcadian landscape depicted here has suffered from passing storm clouds in the recent past (with industrial action by physicians), and it might easily acquire permanent darker textures.

1 Reerink E. Improving the quality of hospital services in The Netherlands. The role of CBO: the National Organization for Quality Assurance in the Netherlands. *Quality Assurance in Health Care* 1990;**2**:146–54.
2 Van der Voorde F, Van der Snoek JA, Reerink E. A quality assurance study of the barium enema. *Quality Review Bulletin* 1981;**6**:10–13.
3 Rittersma J, Casparie AF, Reerink E. Patient information and patient preparation in orthognatic surgery. *J Maxillofacial Surg* 1980;**8**:206–9.
4 Dutch Issue: Quality Assurance in The Netherlands. *Australian Clinical Review* 1987; **7**:1–54.

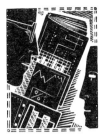

Quality management in the NHS: the doctor's role—I

D M BERWICK, A ENTHOVEN,
J P BUNKER

The doctor and the patient enter the examining room and the door is closed. For even the most jaded doctor and the most cynical patient the click of the door catch creates a special and privileged space. In that space trust can develop, needed disclosures can occur, tears can flow, lifelong burdens can be lifted and explored, and information of the most delicate and significant character can flow from one attentive human being to another. Doctor, patient, and society have conspired to create that space because, in the end, we all need it.

But no door bolts tightly enough to exclude the realities that have come to besiege modern medicine. Doctor and patient can ask for—and have a right to—privacy, but they will not be assured insulation from the times. Real life enters the consulting room through seams and pores. Care costs too much in America, and payers are asking why. They are studying the practice of medicine and manipulating the rules of payment. Studies show levels of variation in clinical practice that offend logic.[1] Patients, made wary by newspaper accounts of malpractice and by their own experience of rushed, insensitive systems, approach formerly trusted doctors with increasing confusion and uncertainty. Doctors, experiencing the unexpected burden of scrutiny and accountability, become unhappy in their work, defensive, and perhaps even emotionally less available to the patients who need them.

To be sure some of these trends have been far more pronounced in the United States and in several western European countries than in the United Kingdom. In the United Kingdom the NHS as a structure has tended to diffuse the anger and anxiety that has come to characterise medical care in the United States. In addition, the cost of health care—the most important single source of pressure on the American system of care—has been maintained in the United Kingdom at a remarkably low level (as a percentage of the gross national product). Health care absorbed 11·8% of the United States gross domestic product in 1989, but only 5·8% in the United Kingdom.[2] Though it has taken its share of criticism for its queues and rationing choices and for the development of a privileged private care market, the NHS remains overall a system that compares favourably to the American system in its commitments to equity of access and cost control.

But the seams of the NHS are worn thin. Expenditures, though rising more slowly than elsewhere, are a matter of increasing political controversy. There are widespread concerns that care is too often delayed, that access to technology is too severely rationed, and that NHS resources have failed to keep pace with needs. Complaints of deficiencies in service levels have become commonplace. It seems unlikely that increases in spending alone can cure this. Moreover, the full potential of truly community based care that the regional and district structure offers has never been fully realised. As in other countries trying to absorb the wonders of high tech medicine, health care in the United Kingdom has become fragmented in its relationships among general medicine; public health medicine; and hospital based acute, largely technical care. A system that would best operate as a seamless whole works instead in functional compartments that leave many patients unhappy and providers of care frustrated. For some even the quality of care provided in the NHS is now seriously in doubt.[3]

NHS reforms

One of us (AE) has suggested that the seeds of poor service, fragmentation, and rising costs were planted in the very structure of the NHS.[4] That structure has survived because of the quality and dedication of the people who work in it and the underlying social commitment to equity, but it lacks strong incentives for the improvement of care and service. In fact, the incentives regarding improvement in the NHS have been perverse: better performance may be associated with higher workload but without a commensurate increase in resources. The widely criticised waiting lists for inpatient surgery are one result.

Recent reforms in the NHS have been directed towards establishing structures and incentives that can encourage quality and efficiency.[5] The reformers of the NHS intend to make it more sensitive to the needs of those who depend on it for service and care and to encourage providers of care to discover better ways to do their work. Under the new rules those who improve their performance would benefit from increased resources with which to handle their expanding share of the medical marketplace.

The central idea is to create incentives for improvement by creating internal "markets" among components of the health care system. Under the new rules the district health authorities become selective purchasers of services that they were formerly obliged to "purchase" only from themselves. It now becomes the duty of the general manager of the district health authority to seek better deals for the patients for whom he has responsibility. With a fixed budget it is in both the patient's and the manager's interest for the authority to contract for services not only at lower prices but with better outcomes, as a poor outcome may necessitate further treatment at additional cost. When the general practitioner is the budget holder it is similarly in his or her interest to contract for the most cost effective care available.

From the perspective of classical economic theory structural reforms based on a market model seem to offer a particularly attractive solution. They suppose improvement to occur as a result of reliable, natural laws of economics in which customers and providers find efficient solutions to their respective needs and constraints. With three basic components—freely available information on the quality of available goods and services, consistent and rational buyers, and competent producers—a market can unconsciously (through the "invisible hand") achieve efficiency and quality levels beyond those attainable by even the most talented planner.

Failures in market conditions of health care

The problem, of course, is that the conditions of an effective market have not been met in medicine. Information by which to judge the quality of medical care is inadequate and has not been freely available to the purchasers of care, whether patients or their agents, insurance companies or the government. Purchasers of care in America, again whether patients or their agents, have been inconsistent and often seem irrational in their demands and expectations. Evidence of variable quality and widespread "inappropriateness" in the medical care of both countries[3] has cast doubt on the competence of the producers of medical care—doctors, hospitals, and others. No one in health care seems to face simultaneously all of the costs and benefits associated with his or her decisions, and there seems to be no market forcing all to make responsible, cost conscious, consistent choices.

The concerns about health care go far beyond worries over the competence of individual clinicians. They are concerns rather about the properties of the system of care—a system in which excess costs and failures in quality can occur despite the best intentions and the best efforts of the people involved.

These imperfections in the medical marketplace are the object of much activity in the United States, and are addressed directly in the plans for a revised NHS in the United Kingdom (while still trying to retain universal, comprehensive services, financed by tax and free at the point of service). In both countries many propose to solve deficiencies in information with more aggressive and sophisticated forms of measurement and publication of the results of care, often using new and powerful computer technology. American payers and regulatory agencies have vastly increased their demands that hospitals release data on their own performance, and in at least some states laws have been passed requiring that hospitals purchase commercial software packages allowing standardised reporting of both the costs and outcomes of care. Recently American doctors have begun to be drawn under the same microscope of performance measurement. In the proposals of the NHS reforms measurements of performance of care givers will also be intensified.

Better information should lead to more consistent and rational behaviour of buyers. The current governmentally supported development and promulgation of standards and preferred practice guidelines in the United States, its sponsors hope, can help to inform a confused public as well as to control the variable practices of the medical profession. In addition, there is renewed interest in financing reforms designed to shift a portion of payment from insurance systems to the pockets of patients themselves, so that the patients become more "sensitive" to the costs of the care they consume and, presumably, therefore consume that care more prudently.

Under the NHS reforms the job of making cost effective and consistent market choices will fall largely on the district health authority and on budget holding general practitioners, whose choices are supposed to reflect priorities among the needs and desires of patients. Purchasing services on behalf of patients is a new responsibility, of which these decision makers have had little previous experience. While there has been some success in the cost effective contracting for care by insurers in America, the obstacles are many and the start up process will be difficult, requiring new data, new data systems, and new skills. Much assistance could be made available, however, from the largely untapped epidemiological and quantitative knowledge of the public health doctors.

Management of care and its quality: the missing link

Better and more widely available information on the outcomes of medical care, together with consistent and rational purchasers, are essential to an effective market, but these alone are insufficient to produce real improvement in quality. For improvement in effectiveness and efficiency to occur the producers of a good or service must also have the capacity to improve performance and to function in a system that facilitates improvement. Of course, if the marketplace is already replete with competent producers working in an optimum system, information and consistent buyer behaviour may achieve a great deal by putting the incompetent out of business—a Darwinian solution to the pursuit of excellence. But when the problems of production are more diffuse—that is, when excellence is not the rule or deficiencies are widespread—then the primary hope of society lies not in selection but in reform. Survival of the fittest will not suffice; the fit must be created.

When the producer is not competent to improve, then available information on quality and lucid purchasers induce only better marketing, not better performance. People tend to limit their attention only to the information and to neglect the need for reform of the products and services the information is supposed to represent. That is exactly what was experienced in the United States when the Health Care Financing Administration (the federal agency that purchases care for elderly people in the United

States) publicly released data on mortality in hospitals across the United States.[6] Instead of rededicating themselves to reducing mortality the hospitals attacked the administration's data and analyses. Seeing no easy way to improve their results, the hospitals spent their energy disputing the accuracy of the information and defending the acceptability of their results.

We contend that, in its current wave of reform, the NHS has a clear opportunity to avoid the errors of policy that have drawn the health care system in the United States into a costly cycle of surveillance, contention, and stagnation. We believe that a focus on measurement and prudent purchasing, though essential steps towards improving the quality and efficiency of the NHS, alone will not be sufficient. What is required in addition is an aggressive plan for strengthening the capability of the various components of the NHS to improve the processes of their own work. Physicians must play a central part in the development of that capability, acquiring, in one sense, a new set of "clinical" skills, equipping them to be physicians to the system in which they work as well as to the individual patients who rely on that system.

Agenda for improving management of care

Our proposed approach rests largely on the experiences of industries outside health care that have faced an urgent need to improve. It was the Japanese, challenged by the massive task of postwar industrial reconstruction, who led the way in applying the principles of management that have since come to be called "continuous quality improvement" or "total quality management" (TQM). Taught largely by American experts sent to Japan to help in the 1950s, Japanese manufacturers developed their skills in making products and services that could better satisfy their customers. The result is international economic history. In many areas of production Japanese firms have acquired worldwide dominance in the past two decades, forcing the developed countries of the West to re-examine their own approaches to management.

In more recent years several American and European firms have become expert in the methods of TQM and have begun to reap the same results as the Japanese. Early concerns that "quality management" was, in its essence, bound to the cultural circumstances of Japan have now been allayed as Western firms, too, have used the methods to their own advantage with Western workforces.

The principles of TQM are not arcane, but neither are they obvious to those schooled in classic general management. The theoretical background of TQM reaches deeply into several disciplines: industrial engineering, social psychology, statistics, and systems theory, to name a few. At its core, TQM relies on four general theses: firstly, that organisational success depends fundamentally on meeting the needs of those it serves (its "customers"); secondly, that quality (defined as the ability to meet the needs of the customers) is an effect caused by the processes of production, in which the causal systems are complex but, with effort, understandable; thirdly, that most human beings engaged in work are intrinsically motivated to try hard and to do well; and, fourthly, that simple statistical methods, linked with careful collection and analysis of data on work processes, can yield powerful insights into the causal systems within processes, on the basis of which those processes can be improved.[7-11]

Management in the TQM world is guided by these four basic notions, the implications of which are challenging to many prevailing beliefs about the best ways to lead organisations. As most workers are presumed to be trying hard most of the time, for example, the TQM approach places little reliance on incentives and exhortations to encourage people to try harder or to do better. "They are already trying," says the practitioner of TQM, "and so how much can be gained by imploring them to try harder?" Instead, TQM theory directs attention not at the workers, but rather at the processes of work in which those workers are bound. Most flaws come from processes, not people, and it is the duty of managers and leaders to assure that those processes are designed and improved so as to permit the "willing workers" to do what they already want to do—their very best.

TQM seeks improvements not by simply measuring results and offering feedback. If processes of work are the sources of excellence or flaw, then the road to improvement lies in deepening knowledge about the causal systems within those processes. In medicine the process of patient care, as it would be defined in the context of TQM, includes administrative procedures by which care is brought to the patient as well as the diagnostic and therapeutic procedures themselves. That breakdown in administrative procedures can cause serious damage to patient care is well known to clinicians but has been largely ignored in quality assurance programmes. The figure gives examples of how such breakdowns can be identified and analysed.

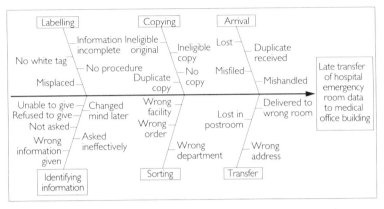

Cause and effect diagram composed from data from national demonstration project on quality management in health care.[12] Issue of interest was timely transfer of hospital emergency room data to satellite medical office buildings. Some 24 theories were advanced by the team. Understanding these interrelations allowed the team to design tests and collect data to confirm or rule out the hypotheses.

The manager of TQM becomes a doctor to the work process. Just as a doctor listens to the patient's symptoms and engages in scientific inquiry to understand the causes behind those symptoms, the manager in a TQM environment "listens to" the work processes—the patterns of success and failure—and, through disciplined use of a scientific cycle of data collection, analysis, hypothesis formation, and hypothesis testing, gradually introduces changes in those processes designed steadily and forever to improve their ultimate performance—their "quality" in meeting customer needs.

TQM goes a step further in suggesting that the scientific method for the improvement of work processes need not be the work solely of managers and executives. As has been proved time and again in manufacturing companies, even workers at the lowest levels of formal education and skill can be taught to use simple statistical methods in their own approach to their own, local process of work. This "democratisation of science," as Professor George Box has called it, can give an organisation enormous leverage towards improvement. Mature quality management organisations of several thousand employees can have at any one time hundreds of process improvement teams at work, involving most employees actively in the step by step improvement of their own work methods.

218

This widespread deployment of improvement requires investment by organisations in the continuous education of all of their employees. Workers in such companies spend weeks each year learning and refining their skills in statistical thinking, crossfunctional cooperation, and awareness of the real needs of external and internal customers. In addition, managers in these environments must pay special attention to potentially toxic aspects of the organisational culture that can inhibit learning and sharing of information. "Drive out fear," counsels W Edwards Deming, one of the leaders of the modern quality revolution, as one of his famous "fourteen points for top leaders."[8] If people are afraid of each other within an organisation, if information can be used to harm someone, or if managers blame people for failures built into the processes of work, then real quality improvement can easily grind to a halt. Information is withheld, functional areas retreat into their own walls, and people seek safety instead of learning. Reducing fear and apprehension in the TQM world is a job for leaders.

Most importantly, TQM entails a steady search for opportunities to improve, even in systems that historically function at satisfactory levels. In a TQM organisation people do not ask "Did I pass inspection?" but rather, "How could I do this better?". TQM rejects reliance on inspection to improve quality and it equally rejects minimalist "pass or fail" standards of performance. Inspection of final results and scrapping of rejects is a costly way to overcome failings in a production process, and alone it offers little knowledge about the underlying causes in the processes that caused those results. Standards—especially minimalist standards that seek to sort the acceptable from the unacceptable—tend to lead to defensive behaviours and tend to quell the search for improvement in the vast majority of those who are being judged.[13] If the "standard" for postoperative infection rates is, say, 2·0% then people tend to spend their time trying to get their rates just below that level. Those whose rates are 1·0% have little incentive to find a way to make them even better. The result is mediocrity, or at least missed opportunities for improvement.

Can total quality management help in health care?

Methods of management that have developed in manufacturing environments are naturally regarded with scepticism in nonmanufacturing settings. The service industries in general have been slow to learn and adopt TQM methods, although in recent years major advances in service quality management have begun to occur.

The scepticism of health care leaders towards TQM has been even greater. Many of the basic principles of TQM are difficult to translate directly into the medical world.[14] For example, how can medicine adopt meeting the needs of the customer (patient) as its driving purpose when so many patients do not seem to know their own needs? Indeed, there is a widespread (but not well documented) opinion in America that many patients demand tests, treatments, and procedures that their doctors know will not help them.

Furthermore, what about the notion that processes not people are the sources of quality and defects in quality. Surely when errors occur in medicine it is more often than not the doctor—a person—who is the underlying "cause." How can we assert that improvement in medicine requires attention to "processes of work" when everyone knows that deficient doctors can cause so much trouble?

The corrosive effects of fear and apprehension on improvement are all too visible in public systems like the NHS. As the object of continuous political debate the NHS must answer daily for its performance, including explaining undesirable events that inevitably arise in complex systems. TQM requires an open, honest search for errors and inefficiencies, which are, in fact, opportunities for improvement. This openness seems at best naive and at worst suicidal when the same information can readily be converted into a weapon used to attack the discoverer of the flaw, the discoverer's institution, and the Ministry.

Most of all, how can medicine afford to tackle "continuous improvement" at a time in history when its resources must be constrained. Quality costs money; everyone knows that. And there will be in the medicine of the 1990s not more money, but less, relative to demands.

Doctors and managers in a few pioneering health care organisations (for example, Henry Ford Health Systems, Detroit, Michigan; SSM Health System, St Louis, Missouri; Park Nicollet Medical Center, Minneapolis, Minnesota; and West Paces Ferry Hospital, Atlanta, Georgia[15]) are beginning to discover that these concerns about the applicability of TQM to medicine may rest more on myth than on fact. "Meeting customer needs," they think, is not at all a bad definition for health care quality, and organisations that wish to remain effective and proud in a time of declining resources must be increasingly precise in understanding exactly what those needs are, including knowledge of the degree to which medical interventions restore or preserve health status. Patients, these organisations believe, have sensible, understandable, reasonable expectations of health care, by and large, and they become distressed, and rightly so, when health care systems fail to meet such basic requirements as answering questions, providing access, and easing pain.

Rising costs, these health care organisations think, may reflect the absence of quality in processes of work. Flawed processes produce a great deal of wasted effort, duplication of effort, and complexity, and they perform unpredictably, leading to frustration among both customers and workers. In manufacturing the costs of poor quality (waste, duplication, unreliability, and so on) routinely have amounted to 25–40% of the costs of production before TQM. Those industrial quality experts who have begun to venture into medical organisations to help them are reporting costs of poor quality just as high, or even higher.[16–18]

The more those innovative organisations understand the causes of poor quality, the richer have become their notions of where flaws arise and why. Surely some defects in care are, in fact, traceable to the doctor, and the doctor alone (medicine has its share of troubled and inept people at work), but, it turns out, the causes of most failures of care are not explained at all by appealing to the myth of "doctor as cause." In health care, as in other complex production systems, quality fails often despite the best efforts of the people who are trapped in the processes of work. As George Labovitz has said, in health care, as elsewhere, quality fails not because people are doing the right thing wrong, but because they are doing the wrong thing right.

One hospital's associate medical director, who is committed to learning and using TQM methods, likes to recount a conversation he had with a receptionist in his own internal medicine unit. Wanting to learn more about local processes of work, the doctor spent an hour at his receptionist's side, watching her perform a long list of pressing tasks. The tasks looked endless and frequently conflicted with each other, but the receptionist struggled gamely through them.

"Your job seems impossible to me," said the doctor, "No one can really do it right."

"I know that," replied the receptionist, "I just try to do my best. It helps to be philosophical about it."

"But, who designed the job this way?" asked the puzzled doctor, "Don't they know any better?"

The receptionist paused, embarrassed, for a moment, and then said sheepishly, "You did, doctor. You did."

Often "the wrong thing" happens not within single functional areas—like medicine, nursing, pharmacy, or administration—but rather at the boundaries or interfaces among functions. In health care staff and organisations remain largely bound in well fenced functional subdivisions or compartments, making it easy for people to blame each other (doctors blame nurses, nurses blame technicians, one department blames another) and difficult for any of them to see the processes of work as a whole—the way the patient experiences it. In technical terms medicine, like oldstyle manufacturing, has tended to suboptimise functions at the expense of its customers and at high financial cost. This lesson applies as well to the modern hospital as it ever did to the factory production line.

In a demonstration project applying TQM methods in the University of Michigan Hospitals one team was assigned to examine reasons for delays in patient discharges, which resulted in delayed access to beds for new patients. Because it was cross functional in its make up, involving doctors, nurses, clerks, and technicians who otherwise rarely talked with each other, the team was able to discover multiple misunderstandings among departments, whose smooth cooperation was logically necessary to the proper functioning of the "discharge process." With simple clarifications of tasks and needs, and with deepening knowledge of how the discharge process really worked, the team was able to shorten the average time new patients spent in the admissions area awaiting an available hospital bed from 3·1 hours to 21 minutes. To achieve these gains required not a penny of additional resources—only new understandings among interdependent functional groups.[12]

The experience of process failure is frustrating and demoralising for people at work. Those symptoms—frustration and low morale—are seeping into health care widely today. The early practitioners of TQM in health care think they understand a good deal about why that is occurring. Health care is frustrated because it has not learned how to get better. TQM, with its emphasis on continually improving the overall process by which we administer care, offers a plausible mechanism. Indeed, we have already taken the first step in our attempts to set standards or guidelines for the process of medical care. It has even been recognised that standards will have to be regularly reviewed and updated on the basis of new knowledge. When this process of review has been accepted and incorporated into practice, and when we have expanded the review of process to include processes of the organisation and delivery of care, as we discuss in the second part of this article, we will have achieved TQM.

Modern medical care is a complex enterprise entailing interactions among doctors, nurses, and other health professionals: complex information systems; an immense array of pharmaceutical products; and complex devices, equipment, and rules of procedure. For good results these complex elements must be assembled effectively, and improvement depends on the processes of care and management that orchestrate these many elements. Such orchestration is not easy. The NHS reforms are designed to increase the freedom and willingness of hospitals to identify and seize opportunities for better coordinating of the elements of care. TQM is a method for achieving just that.

1 Wennberg JE, Gittelsohn A. Variations in medical care among small areas. *Sci Am* 1982;**246**:120–34.
2 Schieber GJ, Poullier JP. International health spending: issues and trends. *Health Affairs* 1991;**10**:106–16.
3 Bunker JP. Variations in hospital admissions and the appropriateness of care: American preoccupations? *BMJ* 1990;**301**:531–2.
4 Enthoven AC. *Reflections on the management of the National Health Service: an American looks at incentives to efficiency in health services management in the UK.* London: Nuffield Provincial Hospitals Trust, 1985. (Occasional paper 5.)
5 Secretaries of State for Health, Wales, Northern Ireland, and Scotland. *Working for patients.* London: HMSO, 1989. (Cmnd 555.)
6 Berwick DM, Wald DL. Hospital leaders' opinions of the HCFA mortality data. *JAMA* 1990;**263**:247–9.
7 Juran JM, Gryna FM Jr, Bingham RS Jr. *The quality control handbook.* New York: McGraw-Hill, 1979.
8 Deming WE. *Out of the crisis.* Cambridge, Massachusetts: MIT Center for Engineering Study, 1986.
9 Feigenbaum AV. *Total quality control.* New York: McGraw-Hill, 1961.
10 Imai M. *Kaizen: the key to Japan's competitive success.* New York: McGraw-Hill, 1986.
11 Scholtes PR. *The team handbook.* Madison, Wisconsin: Joiner Associates, 1988.
12 Berwick DM, Godfrey AB, Roessner J. *Curing health care: new strategies for quality improvement.* San Francisco: Jossey-Bass, 1990.
13 Berwick DM. Controlling variation in health care: a consultation with Walter Shewhart. *Med Care* 1991;**29**:1212–25.
14 Berwick DM. Commentary: peer review and quality management: are they compatible? *Quality Review Bulletin* 1990;**16**:246–51.
15 Walton M. *Deming management at work.* New York: GP Putnam's Sons, 1990:83–117.

16 Batalden PB, Buchanan ED. Industrial models of quality improvement. In: Goldfield N, Nash DB, eds. *Providing quality care: the challenge to clinicians.* Philadelphia: American College of Physicians, 1989:133–55.
17 Berwick DM. Continuous improvement as an ideal in health care. *N Engl J Med* 1989;**320**:53–6.
18 Laffel G, Blumenthal D. The case for using industrial quality management science in health care organizations. *JAMA* 1989;**262**:2869–73.

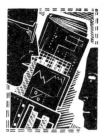

Quality management in the NHS: the doctor's role—II

D M BERWICK, A ENTHOVEN,
J P BUNKER

We have argued that the introduction of market conditions into the NHS, designed to achieve greater accountability and create incentives for efficiency and improved quality of care, will not alone be sufficient to achieve improvement.[1] Also needed is a sound and effective method by which medical leaders, managers, and practitioners can implement strategies for improvement. In the absence of such a method efforts to reform the financing of medical care and increases in accountability may result in more waste and fear than in progress.

We propose that total quality management (TQM), a collection of approaches to quality, efficiency, and leadership that has matured over the past few decades in industries other than health care, can be used effectively within the health care system as a powerful force for improvement. Last week we reviewed basic principles of TQM and suggested how, with appropriate modifications, these principles can apply to the work of medicine; how market forces can increase the motivation for improvements in quality and efficiency; and how TQM can provide a method for acting on that motivation.

In this chapter we explore the special opportunities that TQM offers to NHS doctors as leaders of a partnership of managers and other health professionals who together share stewardship of health care in Great Britain. For this partnership of doctors and managers to be effective it will be necessary that doctors understand and participate in management decisions and that managers understand and contribute to the formulation of the goals of medical care.

To achieve fundamental improvement in care new skills will be needed by doctors and managers. These include the ability to work in interdisciplinary teams; to understand medical care as a continually changing and updated process; to collect and interpret data on patient needs, satisfaction, and values, as well as outcome; to accept the need for and take advantage of the opportunities presented by new methods for the drafting, revision, and implementation of standardised patient care management plans or protocols; to collect, aggregate, and analyse and interpret data on the processes of care; and to facilitate the exchange of information with patients. Finally, most important of all is the need for leadership among doctors and managers.

Doctor's essential role in total quality management

If TQM is to succeed in health care, as we think it can, then doctors will have to have a central role in its practice. This applies even more fundamentally to the NHS than to the disaggregated, fee for service American medical economy. Put boldly, the NHS, unlike much of American health care, is, or at least can be, a system, and because of that it has great potential for rational planned action to meet the needs of those it serves. But that systemic property also creates strong and ineluctable bonds among its components, no one of which can act without the participation of all the others.

The doctors of the NHS, specialists and generalists alike, are key parts of that potential system, and its success may rise or fail depending on the willingness of British doctors to learn, accept, and adapt to the new circumstances of work in an integrated system of care. We believe that TQM offers a set of general principles with which the British medical profession can build an NHS of the future that is proud, capable, supported by its constituents, and, indeed, as satisfying to work in as it has been in the past.

To achieve this transformation will require that doctors accept a body of new skills to learn and practice. Though not taught in medical school, these skills are essential for proper work in an interdependent system of care. Indeed, so crucial are these skills to the successful conduct of medicine in the future that we suggest they be classified as the "new clinical skills" of modern, integrated medical care. They belong in the repertoire of the doctor just as much as the "classical clinical skills" that the new system must preserve and support.

"New clinical skills" of quality management

The "new clinical skills" are as follows:

(1) The ability to perceive and work effectively in interdependencies

Doctors can and should bear ultimate responsibility for much that occurs in clinical patient care. But it is no longer true, if it ever was, that important patient care processes occur mostly in the transactions between one doctor and one patient. Almost all complex care and much of the care that is simple requires faithful, clear, mutually respectful collaboration among workers with many different credentials. In TQM terms most key processes in health care are cross functional.

For cross functional processes to work in the best interests of those served by them the internal dependencies within those processes must be carefully and explicitly cultivated. On assembly lines workers in TQM organisations learn to ask each other such questions as, "What exactly do you need from me in order to do your work properly?" and "How have I done at meeting your needs?" These internal "customers and suppliers" seek to clarify their mutual needs and constraints so as to serve each other better.

In a TQM hospital it would be customary for surgeons to approach sisters on the wards regularly with the question, for example, "Is there anything I could have done last week that would have made your work easier?" Teams would exist in which people involved in a common process—such as ordering and reporting laboratory test results, or controlling postoperative pain, or the registration of patients for hospital admission—would take the time to meet, to make their processes or work explicit through such techniques as flow diagrams, and to plan specific steps towards process improvement. In such teams hierarchy, education, and status would count for little compared with knowledge of the processes and a willingness to contribute ideas.

How would most doctors fare in a culture that self consciously tried to clarify and manage interdependencies like these? No doubt doctors are as ready as others to listen and share ideas, but traditional medical roles and hierarchies of status may place barriers before doctors who wish to attempt better cross functional work. New skills are needed: the skills and willingness to listen across professional boundaries, to remain silent so that others of different status or background as well as one's colleagues can speak, and to realise that the idea of "process" is a great equaliser. In improving processes degrees and rank matter little; what matters are commitment, knowledge, an open mind, and, perhaps, a little humility.

(2) The ability to work in teams

A corollary of awareness of interdependency is the willingness to work effectively in teams, to share responsibility, and to relinquish absolute professional autonomy in the service of a shared purpose. TQM entails in most mature models the creation and activity of numerous specially formed teams of people who together can understand and experiment with processes in a way that no one person or no one function can. Teamwork takes time. Effective teams in health care will in almost all situations require active participation of doctors and frequently their leadership. Yet many doctors seem uncomfortable with real team activity. Where TQM has been tried in hospitals so far doctors are often not effective on quality improvement teams. They arrive late or not at all to meetings; they dominate when they are present; and they some-times leap to solutions before the team has done its proper diagnostic work on the process. They do with processes what they would rarely do with patients—assume that they have the answer even before the question has been clearly formulated and data have been collected. If working in teams is an essential new skill in clinical medicine then it belongs in the curriculum and conscious-ness of medical education at all levels.

(3) The ability to understand work as process

Work should be understood as a process that is subject to continuous review and improvement as new and better data become available.

Effective management of quality begins with deepening under-standing of the actual way in which work is done, and this exploration requires disciplined methods and an open mind. For the doctor in TQM the key question when something goes wrong is not, "Who did this?" but rather, "What is the underlying process of work that contains the likely causal system?" Becoming process minded is harder in medicine than in other industries, largely because so much of the way work is done in medicine has been inherited and not consciously designed.

Note that the term "process" in the TQM context has a more inclusive meaning than is usual in medical contexts. In health care "process" usually refers to clinical care. In TQM it means the way in which work is done, and it refers to work sequences of any type, clinical, non-clinical, or the interface between these two.

An orientation towards understanding processes or work is an important first step towards "driving out fear," one of the central precepts of TQM. The fear to be driven out in medicine is the fear of being made the scapegoat, of appearing to be ignorant, or just of looking foolish (and even, increasingly, of being sued for malpractice). It is a fear that leads to efforts of concealment. When one blames processes and not people it becomes safer to lay bare the relevant facts and for everyone to get to work to improve the process. Angry, accusatory behaviour by doctors who are frustrated by poor results may give those doctors a good deal of self satisfaction at the moment but will be unlikely to result in fundamentally better performance in the long run. On the other hand, seeing work in process terms can easily lead the physician and everyone else to understand that "there, but for the grace of God, go I" and results in the sort of empathetic and collaborative behaviour that fosters improvement. How silly it is to blame people for process flaws.

(4) Skill in collecting, aggregating, analysing, and displaying data on outcomes of care

Quality improvement requires the collection and analysis of data on patient needs, patient satisfaction, and patient values and preferences, as well as data on outcomes. These are types of data with which physicians have had little experience.

There is an important linkage between the measurement of health status outcomes and patient satisfaction, on the one hand, and TQM on the other. Outcomes and satisfaction are results, and any organisation or physician interested in improvement must certainly measure results systematically; otherwise how could it navigate? If TQM becomes the way of the future for the NHS then NHS doctors need to become not just accepting of, but enthusiastic about, measuring the results of care. Furthermore, as no single doctor's experience will be sufficient in volume to permit sound inferences about outcomes, doctors must become generous and skilled in contributing carefully collected data on results to common databases, so that the effects of various approaches can be better understood. The purpose of such aggregated data is not judgment and discipline of individuals, but rather education and improvement for all. In *Working for Patients*[2] the government has made a strong commitment to the implementation of computerised medical information systems, and in so doing has set the stage for the collection, analysis, and display of the necessary process and outcome data.

Such measurement and learning is not a small undertaking, but reliable methods are becoming available for routine use.[3] Adjustment for differences in case mix is perhaps the most difficult statistical problem. While still imperfect, improved and practical methods are now available.[4] The recent introduction of simple methods (including methods of gathering patients' self reports) for the reliable measurement of dimensions of health status—such as physical, role, and social function; mental health; self perceived health; and bodily pain—provide us with powerful new tools for assessing patient outcome.[3] These functional outcomes should now become as routine and standard as the measurement of physiological variables is today.[5]

(5) Skills in "designing" health care practices

In the atmosphere of surveillance and apprehension that characterises much of health care, protocols and guidelines for clinical practice have been swept up into a contentious rhetoric. Frustrated payers threaten to use uniform standard practice protocols to judge the quality and efficiency of care givers. Doctors and hospitals resist protocols as "cookbook medicine" that threatens the art and autonomy of medical practice. In this battling a simple fact is often overlooked—namely, that careful artisans often use specific plans to guide them in their own work. Builders use blueprints, chefs use recipes, teachers use lesson plans, artists use sketches; and doctors themselves, perhaps not recognising them as such, have used diagnostic and therapeutic routines as "rules of thumb," often handed down from "the chief," for as long as medicine has been practised.[67]

In the improvement of quality specific protocols of action—statements of intended behaviours and practices—can be extremely helpful. Stabilising a procedure is a precondition to improving it.[8] If a cardiovascular surgeon reinvented the process for cardiopulmonary bypass every time it was to be used operations could not proceed smoothly. A paediatrician who fundamentally reconsiders the right approach to the initial treatment of asthma for every single new routine case would be wasting time.

The threat to doctors from protocols arises not from the idea of protocols, but rather from their potential misuse. Used properly, well considered "standard procedures" can improve quality, reliability, and efficiency without compromise in the pride or authority of those who use them.[6] Doctors intrigued with TQM will wish to learn methods for drafting, revising, and implementing some standardised patient care management plans, often called algorithms, protocols, or guidelines. For these doctors such algorithms will serve as blueprints serve builders or as experimental protocols serve researchers. Used in this way care algorithms will not offend the doctors; they will be a tool for learning and improvement.[9]

(6) Skill in collecting, aggregating, analysing, and displaying data on processes of work

Measuring important variables within processes is often even more difficult than measuring outcomes, but it, too, can be done if people have enough commitment and trust in its importance. "Key process characteristics," those aspects of processes of work that relate most closely to achieving desired results and to satisfying customer needs, are part of the measurement system of any mature quality management organisation. Unaccustomed as health care organisations are to measuring outcome systematically, they are even less familiar with process measurement, and yet without process measurements assessing outcomes is simply an exercise in frustration. It is like measuring football scores without any knowledge of the way the game was played—useful for awarding trophies, perhaps, but useless in achieving improvements.

The process of clinical decision making has, of course, not been neglected. Medical audit and its many variants, the measurement of clinical appropriateness, the setting of standards and guidelines, consensus conferences, and clinical algorithms have been the focus of a vast American industry that has had virtually no impact on the quality of care,[10] for reasons we discuss below. The process of how medical care is delivered to patients, a process that can have important impact on patient outcome as well as on patient satisfaction, has been largely ignored.

Health care can borrow from other industries simple methods for measuring and displaying the characteristics of the processes of work that it intends to improve. The basic tools of quality improvement include simple graphical methods like flow diagrams, histograms, and run charts, as well as more complicated methods like control charts, that can help anyone with minimal training understand the nature of variation in the system under study. These graphical tools, as well as a positive view of the role of measurement of both outcomes of care and processes of work, should become part of the "clinical" armamentarium of doctors from medical school onward.[8]

(7) Skills in collaborative exchange with patients

In the TQM approach purpose comes from those served—that is, the customers. All modern practitioners of TQM seek continuous refinement of their ability to know what their customers want and need. They develop and use many ways to find out about those needs and to determine how closely their performance is meeting those needs. Anything produced that does not meet a need is, by definition, waste and poor quality. Efficiency is the ability to meet needs without waste.

This driving core for TQM—meet the needs of those who depend on you—implies a level of dialogue and shared authority that is not customary in medical practice. Patients have become used to a passive role, accepting the advice of doctors without inquiry into their own, special needs. Doctors have become comfortable with assuming that they already know the needs of patients, or can better judge what the patients really want than can the patients themselves. Barry *et al* have recently suggested that much waste and miscommunication occur in the gap between unexpressed patient preferences and the misunderstood intents of doctors.[11] Often, for example, the patient with prostatism is able, with help, to disclose a very different set of relative preferences for, say, operative risks and relief of obstructive symptoms than the doctor may assume. Without sound information on risks, benefits, and preferences the doctor and patient may together make a choice that neither would make with more complete information.

Good doctors often begin encounters with patients with the question, "What can I do for you?" The challenge in TQM is to broaden that question into an organisational and personal way of life, and to ask always not just, "What can I do for you?" but also, after the fact, "How well have I done for you?" Doctors, like all members of the health care team, need training and support to learn to ask these questions, unafraid, in many ways and in many settings.

(8) Skills in working collaboratively with lay managers

One of the most costly side effects of increasing frustration in modern health care has been the estrangement of doctors from the lay managers. In America the matter approaches damaging levels. Medical staff in hospitals spend an extraordinary amount of their formal and informal time criticising, doubting, and questioning the motives of lay administrators. "They do not understand medicine," say the doctors.

Administrators, in their turn, fret about the doctors, who do not seem to be "controllable," or willing to behave realistically given organisational constraints. Many managers count their week successful if the brushfire arguments between doctors and administrators have been kept under control. Little energy is left for collaborative improvement.

In the United States, though much less in the United Kingdom, the conflict between medicine and management has taken another turn as a new breed of doctor-manager, some with bilateral credentials, has taken form. These often talented and highly qualified people live a complicated life, sometimes doubted by colleagues on both sides, each assuming that the chimera's real loyalty lies with the other. Such a breed of doctor-manager seems still to be rare in the United Kingdom.

The conflict is as silly and costly, and TQM has little patience for it. The patients and the other customers of health care could hardly care less about the internal feuds and squabbles. It is not unlikely that most patients and other health care customers imagine that doctors in their meetings spend their time and energy trying to figure out how to make care better, and that managers in their meetings do the same. These same customers might be distressed to learn that their money and the time of professionals of both types was often being consumed in tribal rituals of preparation for war.

TQM will not thrive if this gap persists. Care in modern medicine is complicated, and it crosses over and back between clinical and administrative domains without regard to the sensibilities and treaties between doctors and managers. Collaboration is required if processes are to be improved.

The skill base for such collaboration entails considerable knowledge by each party of the work of the other. Both must be willing constantly to reconsider and potentially to change longstanding habits, assumptions, and processes of work. Lay managers must be made welcome in the clinicians' lair, and clinicians must be helped to understand and respect the many sciences of management. For the collaboration to succeed it is equally important that managers know a great deal about the history of medicine in general, and of the NHS in particular. They must acquire a working knowledge of the conditions under which doctors make decisions by regular visits to the wards and clinics. They must understand the high stakes and uncertain scientific base on which many medical decisions must be made; and to do this they must study the systematic methods used to evaluate medical care: cost-benefit analysis,[12] randomised clinical trials, decision analysis,[13] and outcomes management,[5] including risk adjusted measures management.[4] For them to collaborate effectively with doctors and nurses in the many management decisions that must be made, indeed, to be able to communicate with health professionals, these skills will be essential.

Doctor-managers and consultant leaders

Joint degree programmes can clearly help in fostering collaboration between managers and health professionals, but the familiarity and respect must extend deeply into both professions, and the solution must not be left to depend on the few who bridge the gap themselves through their own career choices. Doctor-managers, if they are to be effective, face the awesome need to be skilled in both of the areas of their responsibility, and to be recognised as having these skills. It is particularly important that they be recognised as leaders in the practice of medicine, for only then will their colleagues accept their leadership and delegate many of the critically important managerial and administrative decisions that profoundly effect how medicine can be practised. If this sounds like a hopelessly utopian goal, this is one area where there has been considerable success in America. Particularly notable is the Robert Wood Johnson Clinical Scholar Program that provides two or three years of support to young doctors, usually on completion of formal residency training, and which has consistently attracted outstanding applicants. Training of clinical scholars varies at the discretion of the individual but focuses predominantly on medical economics, statistics, information sciences, and medical sociology. Graduates of the programme have gone on to accept major positions in medical groups, teaching hospitals, and government.

It will not be enough simply to have a small number of highly trained and talented doctor-managers. Practising general practitioners and consultants will need to have some managerial and quantitative analytical skills. General practitioners, to fulfil their responsibilities as gate keepers and care givers, must understand decision analysis and probability theory. They must be able to take advantage of computerised medical information technology and its access to data relevant to the patient at hand in order to refine the decision whether to refer or to provide care, and if they are going to provide care which treatment will provide the highest probability of the desired outcome. For this to happen it will, of course, be necessary to undergo a level of training not usual in the past, a level of training and expertise perhaps as demanding as that of the specialist consultant.

The consultant leader's need for managerial and quantitative skills are equally great. It is to the clinical leader that we must now turn in meeting the urgent challenge to improve the quality of medical care. It had been hoped that the results of medical audit and consensus conferences and the introduction of clinical guidelines would be adopted by the profession to improve the quality of practice. This has failed to happen, and it is only with clinical leadership that this is now beginning to occur.[14]

The clinical leader must be exactly that, a leader of clinicians, recognised as such by them. He or she must be extremely competent in collaboratively reviewing clinical practices and agreeing on common guidelines according to which clinical decisions will be made. Such a clinical leader must have the managerial and quantitative skills necessary to "manage" the team of colleagues for whom he or she has accepted leadership. This will certainly require additional training and motivation at the outset, but, with time, such quantitative skills should and will become an integral part of clinical and bedside teaching and practice.

Barriers to participation of doctors in managing quality

At least four important barriers must be overcome if NHS doctors are to acquire and rely on these new clinical skills.

(1) Time

Being involved with TQM takes time—the time to learn the methods, to listen to patients, to work on teams, to collect data on processes and results, and to teach others. Where will doctors, used to being (and appearing to be) very busy indeed, find the time to join in this effort? The barrier may be even more severe for the general practitioner in a singlehanded practice than for the hospital based consultant as the consultant is physically present in the organisation that can first and most readily employ the techniques of TQM. The NHS will have to solve this problem, creating ways and means for doctors to participate within the constraints of their already busy lives.

(2) Territory

TQM methods establish control over work processes, thus enabling those doing the work to carry on with a reduced sense of frustration, waste, and helplessness. Paradoxically, this control by people over their own work is established only when people are willing to see themselves as bound in unavoidable interdependency with others. For doctors (and others), used to some clarity about whose turf is whose, the initial feelings can be of discomfort and loss. The agenda of TQM demands none the less that barriers between functional areas be broken down so that cross functional processes can become more transparent and, eventually, streamlined.

(3) Tradition

Medical practice contains habits that will prove dysfunctional in the world of quality management. Many are subtle unspoken rules about who may speak when and to whom, beliefs of where wisdom

236

does and does not reside, and rituals that waste time and diffuse purpose. The rules of interaction in managing quality must be shaped according to three priorities: the increasing of knowledge about the people served, the increasing of knowledge about the processes of work, and the use of scientific methods for improving work. Habits that impede these three objectives will slow the improvement of quality.

The traditions of behaviour are perpetuated through the actions of formal and informal leaders. In the transition to TQM leaders must examine their own behaviours, and change them if required. Do they, themselves, seek and use information about customers and processes? Do they blame people or focus attention on processes instead? Do they produce fear or apprehension in others? Do they, themselves, use statistical methods to interpret data, and do they reserve time for learning, just as they expect others to? Do they place improvement of quality at the top of their own agenda, and, if so, how would others realise this by observing them? Do they rely on exhortation, incentives, and inspection to improve quality, or do they show in their actions that they believe that the missing element when quality fails is usually not motivation but knowledge?

If the capabilities of the NHS are to change through the use of TQM then the change must begin with its leaders, including managers as well as doctors and other health professionals. These changes must surely involve not only the actual NHS apparatus, but also important activities in the prestigious royal colleges which set the norms of behaviour and priority for so much of British medicine.

(4) Trust

However hopeful TQM may be as a useful approach for increasing the capability of the NHS, only a fool would claim that its promise is certain. It is, all things told, we think, the best bet. No other alternative exists that is on its face value as persuasive, nor that has as consistent and dramatic a track record in other industries. It is a risk worth taking.

But taking that risk will entail a very high degree of consistency of purpose and collaboration among the parties to the NHS. TQM requires learning, experimentation, reliance on others, willingness to be vulnerable, and, above all, leadership. The BMJ's editor reminds us, in agreement with "all the quality gurus . . . that nothing works without a strong commitment from an organisation's leaders."[15] That commitment must be reflected in their time, in their behaviours, in their budgets, and, most of all, in the ways they deal with each other. Without it TQM can have little impact. With it there is little to keep British health care and the NHS from being the example for the world to envy that it has been in the past.

1 Berwick DM, Enthoven A, Bunker JP. Quality management in the NHS: the doctor's role—I. *BMJ* 1992;**304**:235–9.
2 Secretaries of State for Health, Wales, Northern Ireland, and Scotland. *Working for patients*. London: HMSO, 1989. (Cmnd 555.)
3 Tarlov AR, Ware JE, Greenfield S, *et al*. The medical outcomes study: an application of methods for monitoring the results of medical care. *JAMA* 1989;**262**:925–30.
4 Blumberg MS. Risk adjusting health care outcomes: a methodologic review. *Med Care Rev* 1986;**43**:351–96.
5 Ellwood PM. Outcomes management: a technology of patient experience. *N Engl J Med* 1988;**318**:1549–56.
6 Berwick DM. Practice guidelines: promise or threat? *HMO Practice* 1991;**5**:174–7.
7 Eddy DM. Clinical policies and the quality of clinical practice. *N Engl J Med* 1982; **307**:343–7.
8 Berwick DM. Controlling variation in health care: a consultation with Walter Shewhart. *Med Care* 1991;**29**:1212–25.
9 Berwick DM. Commentary: peer review and quality management: are they compatible? *Quality Review Bulletin* 1990;**16**:246–51.
10 Margolis CZ. *Solving common pediatric problems: an algorithm approach*. New York: The Solomon Press, 1988.
11 Barry MJ, Mulley AG, Fowler FJ, Wennberg JW. Watchful waiting vs immediate transurethral resection for symptomatic prostatism: the importance of patients' preferences. *JAMA* 1988;**259**:3010–7.
12 Bunker JP, Barnes BA, Mosteller F, eds. *Costs, risks, and benefits of surgery*. New York: Oxford University Press, 1977.
13 Weinstein MC, Fineberg HV, eds. *Clinical decision analysis*. Philadelphia: WB Saunders, 1980.
14 Lomas J, Enkin M, Anderson GM, *et al*. Opinion leaders vs audit and feedback to implement practice guidelines: delivery after previous cesarean section. *JAMA* 1991;**265**:2202–7.
15 Smith R. Medicine's need for kaizen: putting quality first. *BMJ* 1990;**301**:679–80.

Index

Abdominal pain 14, 28
Accident and emergency deparments 14–15, 54
Action centred leadership 172
Acute abdomen 14, 28
Administrators *See* Lay managers
Adverse patient occurrence 142, 147–149
Algorithms 189–197, 231
Alment Committee 4, 34, 171
American College of Surgeons 146
American Medical Association 5
American Medisgrps system 47
American Society of Anesthesiologists 47, 146
Anonymity 165
Appendicectomy 13
Appointments in general practice 137–138
Appropriateness of care 200–201
Assessment form 179
  content and purpose 180–184
  discussion 184–185
Attitudes 27, 39
  consultants 43, 45–46
Audit analyst 84
  meetings 87–88
  projects 88
  setting up a project 86–87
  workload 87
Audit assistants 75, 91
Audit cycle 27, 28, 174–175
Audit facilitators 91
Audit officers
  background 90
  duties 50
  resources 92
  role and rewards 90– 2
  training 93
Australia 38, 209

Bangladesh 209
Bath Health Authority 147
Behavioural change 27, 28, 208
Belgium 209
Bias 132

Birmingham acute medical unit 53
Birmingham Research Unit 25, 31
Birmingham University 116
Blood pressure screening 138–139
Booking policies 22
Box, George 218
Breast screening questionnaire 160
Brighton Health Authority 58, 99, 142, 149
  medical records 54
Bristol and Weston Health Authority 53
British Medical Association 26, 34, 47
British Medical Journal 26, 237
British United Provident Association (BUPA) 47, 58
Bromley Health Authority 147, 149

Canada 28, 31, 37, 38, 209
Case-mix patient management system 53
Case record retrieval 126, 130–131
Case register 126
CASPE Research 58, 142, 160
CBO, Utrecht 205
Census 164
Centrally imposed audit 29–30
Cervical cytology 110, 138
  clinical quality improvement 192–195
Chest *x* ray examination
  before ECT 12
  preoperative 11, 12
Chesterfield and North Derbyshire Royal Hospital 53
Chronic disease 22, 53, 109, 176
  patient satisfaction 162
Claim forms 110
Clarke, Kenneth 171
Clinical audit 51, 68
  basic 72–73
  committees 70, 72
  confidentiality 76
  educational aspects 69
  implementation 74–75
  methods 72–74

Clinical audit (*continued*)
  participants 71
  planning 71
  responsibilities 69–70
  team 85
Clinical leaders 235–236
Clinical management 13–15, 21,
  189–190
Clinical process performance 197
Clinical quality improvement
  process 190–191
  screening for cervical cancer
    192–195
  specification 195–196
Clinical record review 73
Clinical severity index 46–47
Coding 46, 54, 114
Collaboration
  lay managers 233–234
  patients 232–233
Colonic resection 114
Commitment 238
Communication 74, 124, 153, 156
  doctor-patient relationship 176
Community hospital 19
Compartmentalisation 222
Complexity coding 46–47
Computers 46, 54, 75, 109, 230
  software 58
  statistical packages 166
Confidentiality 76, 81–82, 99, 165
Conflict 76, 233
Consensus conferences 200, 201
Consultant leaders 235–236
Consultants' attitudes 43, 45–46
Consultation
  patients' views 153, 156, 160
  techniques 20
Continuous quality improvement 216
Contractual audit 78, 100, 110
Control of audit 29–30
Coordinators *See* Audit officers
Cost-benefit analysis 234
Costs
  audit 30–31, 80–81
  health care 212
  poor quality 221
Criteria 107
Criterion audit 37–38, 73, 99
  advantages 127
  analysing sample records 125–126
  choice of criteria 123–124
  choice of topic 123
  discussion 126–127

repeat audit 127
Critical incidents 19
Customer audit 29
Cycle of audit 27, 28, 174–175

Data 57, 112–115, 229–230, 231–232
  abstracting 126
  analysis 109, 133
  capture 46
  coding systems 114
  collection 64–65, 131
  defining and recording 107–110
  interpretation 58–64, 65
  presentation 66–67, 134
  retrieval 36, 54
Data Med Computer Systems 54
Deaths
  general practice 21
  hospital 119–120
Decision analysis 234
Definition of audit 68–69, 78
Delay patterns in general practice 19,
  23
Deeming, WE 219
Department of Health 68, 81
Design of health care 230
Diabetes 22, 176
Diagnosis
  coding 46, 54, 114
  delay in general practice 23
Disagreement among doctors 200
Disease registers and indexes 109
District audit advisory committee 70,
  92
  objectives 72
District health authorities 213
District medical audit committee
  55–56
District medical audit implementation
  plan 70
District medical education committee
  172
District nurses 138
Doctor-managers 233, 234–235
Doctor-patient relationship 176
  collaboration 232–233
Drug budgets 110
Dunnfile 58
Dutch health care *See* Quality
  assurance in Netherlands
  hospitals

Ear, nose, and throat department 15

Educational aspects 25, 28, 69, 171–172
  key points 176–177
  learning and audit cycles 174–175
  organisation 172
  programmes 173
Effectiveness of audit 27–28
Electroconvulsive therapy 12
Environment 96
Error checking 133
Evaluation 4
Evaluative clinical sciences 201
External audit 5–7, 11, 29–30

Family health services authority 79, 80
Fear 229
Feedback 26, 134
Focused audit studies 73
Follow up 124
  after surgery 13–14, 47
  cervical cytology 194–195
  sampling 165
Formal hospital audit 11
France 209

General practice audit See also
    Problem solving in general
    practice
  advisory groups 78–83
  alternatives for audit 19
  challenge 18
  contractual 110
  duration of data analysis 109–110
  population denominators 108–109
  protocols 107–108
  sources of data 105–106, 110
  studies 19–23
  topics 36, 82, 106
General pratitioners 55, 235
  fundholders 100, 213
Germany 209
Global audit 74
Guidelines 190, 230
  for audit 34–35

Halo effect 155
Harvard Community Health Plan 190, 192
Health Advisory Service 38
Health Care Financing Administration 215–216
Health status 153, 163
Hernia repair 113

Hospital admission variations
  appropriateness of care 200–201
  medical 199
  problems and solutions 201–203
  surgical 198–199
Hospital audit See also Surgical audit
  clinical management 13–15
  data 112–115
  experimentation and publication 15–16
  formal 11
  informal 10–11
  random case review 116–121
  referrals 15
  procedures and units 11–13
  retrospective case review 129–135
  selecting cases 120
  topics 35
Hospital discharge 118, 222
Hospital In-Patient Enquiry 199
Hounslow and Spelthorne Health
    Authority 68
Hove General Hospital 147
Hyaline membrane disease 13
Hydroxycobalamin injections 138
Hypertension 140

Incentives 97
Incident review 73
Indicators 110
Inflammatory bowel disease 115
Informal audit 10–11
Information 36, 54, 215–216
  access 99
  management needs 99–100
  systems 75, 97
Input 7
Intensive care units 13
Interdependencies 222, 227–228, 236
Internal audit 5–7
International Classification of Diseases 46, 54
Interview questionnaires 157, 158
Introduction of audit 38–39
Investigations 53, 109–110, 118
Italy 209

Japan 216
Joint Commission for the
    Accreditation of Healthcare
    Organisations 146
Joint Working Party on the
    Organisation of Medical Work in
    Hospitals, 34

Key process characteristics 231
King's Fund Centre 44, 201
Korner data 120

Laboratory investigations 109–110
Labovitz, George 221
Landelijke Specialisten Vereniging 205
Lancet 39
Lay managers
  collaboration 233–234
  expectations and needs 99–101
  responsibilities 96–99
Learning cycle 174, 175
Life expectancy 199
Likert scale 162
Local audit 11, 30
Lothian surgical unit 43, 47, 115
  coding system 114

Malaysia 209
Managers *See* Lay managers;
    Doctor-managers
Mandatory audit 30
Market conditions
  failures 213–215
  NHS reforms 212–213
Medical audit 51
  characteristics past and future 94–96
  definitions 68–69, 78
  differentiation from review 122
  industrial model 7
  objectives 25–26
  phases 122
  requirements 39
  terminology 3–4
Medical audit advisory groups
  activities of audit 82
  confidentiality 81–82
  local coordinator 80
  meetings 80
  outcome 82–83
  participation 82
  process 79–82
  reports 82
  resources 80–81
  structure 79
*Medical Audit in the Family
    Practitioner Services* 79
Medical audit papers 178
  attributes 179, 182–183
  content and purpose of assessment
    form 179–184
  discussion 183–184
  suitable projects 179

Medical data index 46
Medical education 173
Medical emergencies 53
Medical Management Analysis System
    145–146
Medical management audit 51
Medical negligence 29, 99, 145
  risk management 101
Medical records 19, 36, 109
  quality 54
  retrieval 126, 130–131
  staff 38
Medical specialties 44, 53, 55
Medicare 80
Meetings 75, 80, 88–89, 119
Mental health 207
Methods of audit 37–38, 52–54, 72–74,
    97–98
  categories 122–123
Methotrexate study 86–87
Monitoring 4
Mortality 114, 118
Myocardial infarction 146

National Academy of Sciences,
    Institute of Medicine 80, 201
National audit 11, 112
National Health Service 4, 220, 226
  costs 212
  deficiencies 212
  Management Inquiry 152
  reforms 212–213, 214–215, 216
  Royal Commission 26, 30, 34
National Institutes of Health, 200
Neoplastic disease 23
Netherlands *See* Quality assurance in
    Netherlands hospitals
Neutrality 165
North Derbyshire District Health
    Authority Audit *See also* Audit
    analyst
  committee 55–56
  coordinator 50–51
  methods 52–54
  objectives 49–50
  outcome 55
  participants 50
  problems 54–55
  structure 50
Nurses 71
Nursing 207

Objectives of audit 25–26
Obstetric unit bookings 22

Occupational health 207
Occurrence screening 73, 99
    development 145–146
    multidisciplinary application 145
    pilot study 147–149
    principles 142
    project 149–150
    United Kingdom 146–147
    validity and reliability 146
Office of Population Censuses and
    Surveys 46
Outcome 7, 35, 74, 124
    data 229–230
    intermediate 7
    management 234
    measures 55, 153
    prediction 113
    patients' views 156
    surgical 47, 113
Outpatients 13–14, 47, 55

Papanicolaou smear, abnormal 192
    algorithm 193
    follow up 194–195
Participation in audit 50, 71, 82
Patients 71, 74, 99
    collaboration 232–233
    dimensions of patient satisfaction
        156
    "ghost" 108
    newly registered 108
Patient satisfaction surveys
    alternatives 153–154
    analysis 166–167
    conduct 165
    judgment of patients 155
    negative assumptions 154–155
    piloting a questionnaire 163–164
    questionnaire design 160–163
    reasons for 153
    reliability and validity 155–156
    sample 164–165
    strategy 156–158
    use of results 157
    variability of response 155, 161–162
Peer review 5, 51, 53, 99, 139
Performance
    clinical process 197
    indicators 110
    level 107
Perinatal necropsy 12
Physiotherapy 139, 207
Population denominators 108–110, 164
Porterfield, John 10

Practitioner 26
Prescribing 20–21, 110
Preventive medicine 21, 138
Problem oriented medical records 19
Problem solving in general practice
    136
    advice 141
    deficiencies and problems 140
    less successful audits 139–140
    successful audits 137–139
Process 7, 8, 35
Processes of work 216, 217–218
    cross functional 227–228
    data 231–232
    failure 221–222
    understanding 228–229
Professional Standards Review
    Organisation (PSRO) 5–6, 26, 31
Prostatism 232–233
Protocols 107, 230–231
PSRO See Professional Standards
    Review Organisation
Psychotropic drugs 20
Publication 15–16 See also Medical
    audit papers

Quality assurance 4
Quality assurance in Netherlands
    hospitals
    committees 206
    health care system 204–205
    future 209–210
    method 206–207
    national policy 208–209
    practice 207–208
    problems in health care 205–206
    resource centres 205, 209
Quality improvement See Clinical
    quality improvement
Quality management See Total quality
    management
Quality of care 8
    papers 178
    performance 197
Quality of life 55, 199
Questionnaires
    background variables 163
    design 160–163
    episode specific 160–161
    piloting 163–164
    reliability and validity 155–156
    self completed v interview 157–158
Quota sampling 164, 165

Radiology 11–12, 14
Random case review
    advantages and disadvantages
        116–117
    lessons and achievements 117–118
    limitation 119
    outcome 118
    participation and meetings 118–119
    selecting cases 120
Random sampling 109, 164
Reciprocal visiting 122
Records See Medical records
Records analyst 38
READ codes 114
Referrals 15, 109, 124, 139
    variations 199
Regional audit coordinator 91–92
Regional primary health care
    committee 44
Regional specialist advisory
    committees 43–44
Regional specialty subcommittees
    audit in general surgery 45–48
    membership 45
    role 44
Regional surgical audit report 47
Repeat audit 127
Reporting results 75, 82
Research papers 178
Resource centres 205, 209
Resources 7, 8, 51, 80–81, 96–97
    management 69, 100
Retrospective case review
    bias 132
    data analysis 133
    errors 133
    extraction of data 131–132
    objectives, criteria, standards
        129–130
    presentation and feedback 134
    sample size 130
    time 132
Review 4–7
    differentiation from audit 122
Risk management 101, 234
Robert Wood Johnson Clinical
    Scholar Program 235
Royal College of General Practitioners
    34
    Birmingham Research Unit 25, 31
Royal College of Physicians of London
    34, 55, 116, 171
Royal College of Surgeons of England
    34, 45–46, 171

Royal Commission on NHS 26, 30, 34
Royal Sussex County Hospital 147,
    149

Sampling 109, 164–165
Scottish mortality study 115
Screening criteria See Occurrence
    screening
Screening results 27–28
Setting up audit
    background and basic princples
        68–71
    implementation 74–76
    methods 72–74
Setting of surveys 165
Severity adjusted analysis 120
Severity coding 46–47
Social sciences 176
South East Thames Regional Health
    Authority 99, 149–150
South Western Regional Hospital
    Medical Advisory Committee 44
Spain 209
Specialities 43
    small 54
Staffing 75
Standards 8, 107
    minimalist 219
State run audit 29
Statistics
    accuracy 55
    computer packages 166
Stroke management 130–134
Structure 7, 8
Subgroup analysis 166–167
Summed scales 162, 166
Surgical audit 57
    coding systems 114
    data collection 64–65
    interpretation and presentation of
        data 58–67
    nature and quality of data 112–114
    outpatient follow up 13–14
    regional speciality subcommittees
        45–48
Surgical operations
    complications 59–61
    perioperative deaths 47, 114, 115
    procedures 58–59
    rates 198–199
    return to theatre 61, 63, 64
Systematic sampling 164–165

Targets 107, 110

Teamwork 228
Terminology 3–4
Territory 236
Time 74, 132, 236
Tonsillectomy rates 198
Topics for audit 35–36
  criterion based audit 123
  general practice 81, 106
Total quality management
  background and principles 216–219
  barriers to participation 236–238
  doctor's role 226
  health care 219–223
  "new clinical skills" 227–234
  poor quality 221–222
Tracer diagnoses 19
Tradition 236–237
Trust 237–238

Unit audit committee 70
United States 26–27, 28, 37, 38, 55,
    80, 146, 209, 214, 233
  agency for health care policy and
    research 200

cost of audit 31
cost of health care 212
Harvard Community Health Plan
    190
hospital admission 199
hospital mortality 215–216
operation rates 198–199
University of Michigan Hospitals 222

Variables 107, 163
  manipulation 166
Vascular surgery 64
Vermont 199
Video 122

West General Medical Services
    Committee 34
West Glamorgan 129
Work *See* Processes of work
Working for Patients 150, 152, 202,
    230
World Health Organisation 4

x ray examination 11–12, 14